'VICIOUS CIRCLES'
BY
DIANE HARRISON

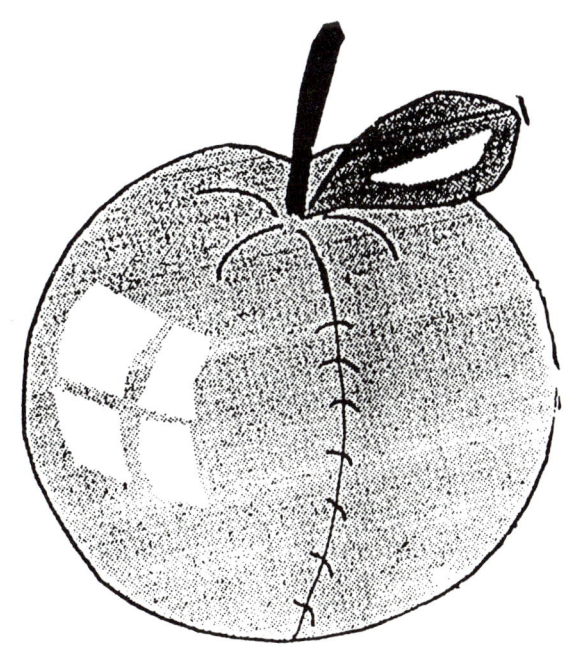

ACKNOWLEDGEMENTS

I wish to thank Sally Gardner for her support and encouragement and Brighton Street Women's hostel. Also Pat and Sal, my friends and colleagues in A.S.H.E.S. training consultancy. Special thanks to Louise Pembroke, Anna, Karin - my manuscript readers and Marc for cooking the tea when I was so engrossed in my work that I lost all sense of time! Lastly I want to send my deepest gratitude to all the women who in some way contributed towards the making of this book. Their courage in speaking out has helped to break the silence surrounding self harm.

DEDICATION

To my children, Mark, Lisa and Rachel Harrison. I am always with you sending my love.

VICIOUS CIRCLES

Contents

		Page No.
	Introduction	2
Section One	WOMEN AND HARM IN CULTURE AND SOCIETY - The roots of conflict	6
Section Two	A FIGHT FOR SELF SURVIVAL - The body as a battleground	18
Section Three	CREATING ORDER FROM CHAOS - A non verbal struggle for expression	38
Section Four	UNDERNEATH THE SKIN - The inner conflict	52
Section Five	TREATMENT AND THERAPIES - Women's experience of help and support	68
Section Six	PERSONAL EXPERIENCES - Journeys of survival	90
Section Seven	RESEARCH FINDINGS	113
Section Eight	SELF HELP - and what has been useful to women Rights for women who self harm.	118
	RESOURCES	128
	BIBLIOGRAPHY	132

INTRODUCTION

I am a survivor of self injury and sexual abuse. I now work as a training consultant on these and other issues related to women's mental health. I am also involved in running groups for women and some individual counselling work. A lot of my time though has been spent in research and writing about self harm because although there are increasing numbers of people coming forward, little is generally known or understood about this issue.

The term 'self harm' can incorporate any number of possible self abusive patterns. These can range from failure to give attention to one's emotional and physical needs, right through to the more direct forms of self laceration or injury through taking toxic substances. Some of the more 'popular' issues are addictions and 'eating disorders' such as anorexia and bulimia which have been written about in some depth by others.

While I will be looking at some of these issues throughout, my main focus is on self inflicted injury, a seemingly frightening and yet quite common act of self abuse. Often called 'shocking' or 'attention seeking' it could best be described as a desperate bid to defend one's own sense of self survival.

This book arises from my own and other women's experiences, which I hope will give you a better understanding of this issue. While I acknowledge this is also an issue for men, I believe that there are certain differences in the way men experience self harm which could be better addressed elsewhere. Nevertheless, I am sure that whoever reads this will recognise something of themselves and will want to question these issues further.

Although it has not been proved conclusively that more women than men are affected, I am looking at issues of power from a woman's point of view: how women are treated, and respond, to cultural, political and social conditioning.

As a woman and a survivor, I have struggled, along with other women, to have my work and ideas taken seriously and to be credited for this. Sometimes in the past, if I have managed to pass my ideas on to clinical or medical staff, I have heard them repeated at a later date by those same people – who then take the credit for them. Or I have seen snippets of my experiences distorted through the media, who try to sensationalise self harm. This reminds me of how women's voices have been silenced, our experiences distorted and our wisdom minimised by those in power who have sought to profit from us.

In the past, powerful women healers were discredited as 'evil' witches or 'madwomen', because, says Ussher, "they challenged the privileged patriarchs, the male experts who believed that a monopoly on healing was their God-given right." Yet they were probably more advanced, at that time than men, says Gage. Women believed in working with the psychological and physical aspects of a person within their environment and were expert midwives and healers using herbs and natural remedies. Since this time, the idea of the whole person has in Western medicine been broken up into different aspects the psychological separate from the physical, which has itself been divided into various pieces.

Similarly, women's experiences of self harm are distorted through others interpreting and misinterpreting their reality until it makes little or no sense. Self harm is treated as a 'dysfunction' of the individual, who is separate from 'normal' society.

Understanding the 'Self' in Harm

Self harm is a broad term used for many various and diverse acts we all use to enable us to cope with the stresses and pain of living.

While we may or may not deliberately harm ourselves, any of these acts (and many more besides) will have some detrimental effect on our long term wellbeing. We may for instance smoke; drink; have problems with food; find ourselves in abusive and otherwise damaging relationships (at home or at work); deny our own needs in favour of others; perhaps worry about how we are seen by the rest of the world. Sometimes we get stuck in rigid beliefs, or hooked into negative thought processes which limit our choices and undermine our true potential. We try to deny the presence of underlying difficulties in our lives because these may seem very formidable. So we stay with what is known and familiar, even if it limits or damages. Generally we are not supported for having personal feelings and find ourselves looking for logical explanations and analyses to justify and make sense of details. So we lose sight of our feelings, which are difficult to verbalise, and their importance is therefore obscured.

Each one of us can in some way reflect the harming society in which we live, where authentic needs are hidden and are kept under some degree of control.

When we look at the many abuses imposed on women and children in society it follows that there are a lot of us who must still carry emotional scars. If we then look at the limited resources and support we have for self expression, what we see are the building blocks of potential harm. We carry our pain in isolation, not daring to share it with another. We fear other people's reactions because we may not be heard by them, so our pain might be belittled or rejected. But most of all we fear our own hurt; we fear finding its depth unsurvivable. So we try to limit the damage by trying to protect ourselves from having to feel these deep, unvoiced hurts. We try to explain them away or seek other outlets.

For instance we might organise our lives so that we have no time to feel anything, or we minimise our own feelings by looking after someone else's problems. Although this may relieve us from having to deal with underlying difficulties in the short term, in time our physical and emotional defences are weakened to such a degree that we become physically and emotionally worn, or 'burnt out.'

I have heard people refer to self injurers as 'not taking responsibility for themselves.' Well maybe those who use that argument should turn it around. When we are acting responsibly we are using whatever experience we already have to make the outcome better or easier to deal with. For example, we would not stay at work after hours, or take work home with us if we were very tired. We might though, if it gained something, or relieved possible pressures. We are acting responsibly by giving thought and care to our work. But when do we stop? What if the pressures continue or escalate? When does working hard become too hard? Maybe if our past experiences in life have been painful, we reflect that pain through our actions to some degree. We may become workaholics, possibly because experience makes us fear non-achievement, not being 'good' enough or overwhelming collapse in our lives. Hard work makes us feel better people, more acceptable to ourselves and to others. Many workaholics go on to suffer from exhaustion, both mental and physical; others suffer from life threatening illnesses. Why should we judge this as being more responsible than the woman who cuts her arm because the pressure of her overwhelming feelings become too much? Who would really wish to harm themselves, whether it be by cutting or less consciously inflicted through overworking unless it seemed the best way of handling life at the time?

That is why this book feels so important. Like many others, I want to encourage more understanding of people who self injure. We have come to accept many other forms of harm such as eating distress and alcohol abuse but as yet, many still describe people who cut their bodies as 'attention seeking'. As if 'manipulatively' causing injury in an effort to gain control of others. I hope readers will pause on their judgments and will look into their own hearts as they move through these pages.

Fear of being well:
No one to look after me
No one to love me
Logic telling me there must
Be a better way.
My battered body yearning for release
From the cuts and poisons.
I see the blood rise
Out of an open wound
To show others
"This is how much it hurts"
A cut, the pain is sweet
Punishment for my neediness.
I smile at the damage
But my body cries for me.
Blood trickles down
– Ruby red tears
Show my sorrows to the world
Sew me up but be gentle
It hurts so much;
The pain in my body
Mirrors that of my mind.

                              Jane 1985

SECTION ONE

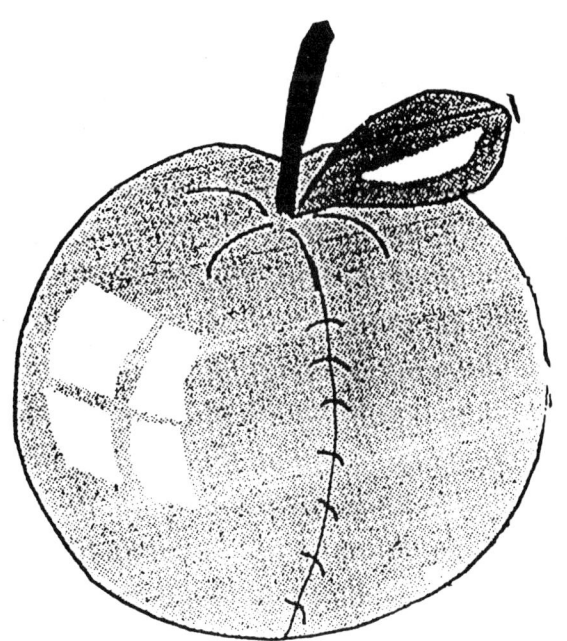

WOMEN AND HARM IN CULTURE AND SOCIETY – the Roots of Conflict

In general women find it harder to show their anger than men, so tend to internalise angry feelings which may result in depression. Men find it more difficult to show their sadness and may redirect their feelings by becoming angry.

This gender issue is important. Women are generally less likely to be taken seriously than men in any sense. We are still lagging far behind men when it comes to being able to speak out and be heard in our own right. Many women believe that they have little to contribute anyway and even when we rise to positions of power we often feel 'unreal' or 'false', as if playing a part which does not really belong to us.

Historically, the powerful figures in each age of history are all, or are mostly, male. Women only became important if they had inherited title or wealth, or sacrificed themselves to a greater cause (Joan of Arc). Look at our history through Art: our great painters (male) depict women in their paintings in submissive positions, often sitting or lying down. Women may adorn a standing male whose status is portrayed by his higher and more dominant position in the picture. Women's importance has decorated a very male picture of life, her attractiveness adding colour but fading with age within the male belief system. The age issue is still important, perhaps even more so in today's throw away society. While a man becomes 'distinguished' with age, an ageing woman becomes a figure of contempt to be hidden or remoulded back into youthful form. I do add, however, both sexes fare badly around age in terms of being accepted as capable human beings.

Every time we switch on the T.V., pick up a paper or magazine, we see beautiful, young and slim women adorning the pictures. Larger or older women usually feature in less important roles such as someone's mother, housekeeper or aunt, the domineering wife, a figure of fun or contempt. It is hard to believe that our living, growing, feeling and ageing selves are natural; that age may bring maturity and wisdom and that this is an important part of life and living.

The bedrock of many of our beliefs are fed to us through the media, who are in turn fed by multinational corporations that invest or have shares in the 'popular' press and advertising. Images of how women 'should' live, how we 'ought' to look surge into our lives every day. Naomi Wolf, in her book 'The Beauty Myth' talks about these issues and says particularly of women's magazines, 'They transmit a myth about beauty as the gospel of a new religion. Reading them, women participate in re-creating a belief system as powerful as that of any of the churches whose hold on them has so rapidly loosened.' The need that we should 'purify' ourselves to redeem our 'sins' has been rewritten into our modern culture. It needs us to feel guilty if we do not fit into a size 8 dress and have lines on our faces. Believing this we can be guided back: through constant dieting and self starvation, or plastic surgery to remove bodily fat and flab; painful electrolysis to remove unwanted body hair. The list goes on indefinitely but women are 'consenting' to be 'purged' of their sins, or at least feeling guilty enough to keep on trying.

This beautiful woman image has followed us through the ages and is upheld by manufacturers and anyone who wishes to profit by us believing that we are less valuable if we do not get a better figure; put on a particular brand of make up; use a certain beauty product; get rid of our wrinkles and fat. Our self esteem plunges as we compare ourselves unfavourably to the beautiful images of young and slim actresses flashed across our T.V. screens, or the fashion models seen in women's magazines. Women's self disgust runs as proportionally high in our society as the political and cultural food we are fed, our self esteem as low as the dismissive and hurtful remarks which are made about us. Yet we feel hungry for a love and acceptance which we are unable to find within ourselves. We try and meet them through our bodies, by trying to change how we look, we try to change how we feel.

Historically, we have been encouraged to think of women as being dependent, childlike, and needing an adult male to care for our needs as only 'he' can make us happy. Heterosexual 'marriage' has been upheld as 'normal'.

'Happy family life' messages are fed to us in the adverts. 'Mum', happy with her wash, shrugs as the children come in covered in mud and fills up the washing machine yet again. After making several instant but expensive snacks for hungry children she goes on to cook a delicious meal for her partner and family. She never looks tired and is always immaculate and ready for whatever role she plays. Mother, nursemaid, wife or lover, she happily immerses herself into each job. But the reality is usually very different. She may be out at work all day and has neither time nor energy to prepare a three course meal. She may not be able to afford to – she may be a single parent. Perhaps she is in a very unhappy, abusive relationship and lives in fear. But whatever her reality, the likelihood is that however much she does, whether she achieves every goal she sets out to do or not, she will feel guilty for her perceived failures. She does not feel happy; the day was stressful, everything went wrong; important appointments were missed because one of the kids was ill. Looking into the mirror she sees a pale and tired face staring back at her, her body telling of all the starches and calories that she has managed to consume throughout the day to give her fuel. No, she does not feel like the successful woman she reads about. She feels like a heap, flopped in front of the T.V. trying to escape into some light relief – which turns out to be another fantasy world full of bright illusions, all alien and unknown to her reality. The effect of this adds to her already stressful life which may lead her into feeling powerless to change her situation. Unvoiced feelings of anger and helplessness may cause her to experience depression.

She may turn to the medical profession for support, or at least something to make her feel better. Sadly, she may get no better deal. Doctors may try to prescribe pills (bought from multinational pharmaceutical companies who invest in medical treatments). These do little to change her situation and she ma y become labelled 'depressed', 'emotional' or even 'over emotional'.

The 'hysterical', 'neurotic woman image follows us through our notes making it feel as if our credibility is at stake. And once we have these labels, any future appointments, for whatever problem, can become clouded with a degree of prior judgment. Doctors are often happy to call illnesses 'psychosomatic' and can dismiss their patients' symptoms as 'all in the mind', as if psychosomatic, mind and body experiences were less real and less important than a more easily recognisable and treatable physical illness. A woman in great distress may have drugs prescribed for her without being told about their side effects or long term consequences. Appointments are made with psychiatrists weeks or even months into the future and she has little say as to when this might be. And when women arrive at their appointments nobody seems clear about what might be on offer in the way of support, how this might help, what else might be available and how to go about finding it. Other people seem to make decisions on her behalf, thus reinforcing her feelings of powerlessness.

A friend of mine, Louise, talks about her experience of hospital Doctors; "Sexist and heterosexist attitudes were common from the psychiatric male, white, middle class psychiatrists. Care with make-up and hair style were seen to be clear indications of getting better, and likewise, wanting marriage and children were viewed by some as part of recovery. I know of individuals who have been told that their problems would get easier if they acquired a boyfriend, automatically assuming heterosexuality. Cure and eradication of the aberrant behaviour were the goals. But it felt like my soul would be the price."

Lucy Johnstone in her book 'Users and Abusers of Psychiatry' says "Hospital characteristically responds by an unquestioning reinforcement of the traditional values that led to the problem in the first place. Thus, these women are routinely assigned to programmes of cooking, shopping and sewing, and their progress is measured by how well they do in these activities." "Not believing that they deserve any better treatment, they pass through the psychiatric system without protesting or attracting the kind of attention that has been paid to less common but more dramatic conditions such as schizophrenia."

Hospitals reflect the stereotyped attitudes we have within the larger society. The assumption is that a woman needs a male partner and a family. These are taken as signs of health. Refusal to accept heterosexist values are assumed to be signs of 'disordered thinking'. "Women who are adventurous, competitive, sexually active, independent, who reject the role of wife and mother – to name but a few examples – may all be designated psychiatrically ill" (Ussher 93). So too have I heard from lesbian women complaining of staff trying to 'treat' them for their sexual identity.

But equally, recent work indicates that "women who conform rigidly to the female model as well as those who unambiguously reject it are likely to be labelled psychiatrically ill, is one we cannot ignore" (Ussher 9). So paradoxically, if we conform too strongly to the stereotypical female role, we might also be labelled ill. Chesler agrees, "What we consider 'madness', whether it appears in women or in men, is either the acting out of the devalued female role or the total or partial rejection of one's sex role stereotype." But these values are dismissive of each woman's experience and choice. They state an abnormality in the way women try, sometimes desperately, to describe themselves as individuals. This pathologises a woman's distress by describing it as a 'disorder' or 'syndrome' in an attempt to categorise any number of 'symptoms' within this framework.

In the 19th century, "hysteria assumed a particularly central role in psychiatric discourse, and in definitions of femininity and female sexuality" (Showalter 85). Its vast array of symptoms, including fits, fainting, vomiting, choking, sobbing, laughing and paralysis, became associated with the feminine nature. Women were deemed to be ruled by their wombs and their 'raging hormones'. Interestingly enough, "many women diagnosed 'hysterical' were more independent and assertive than other women in their peer group." (Ussher 93). So what the doctors labelled 'hysterical behaviour' was in fact a reaction to an oppressive society which demanded total passivity in women.

Today's anorexic who rejects our 20th century expectations of women could be one and the same as the 19th century 'hysteric.' Indeed the diagnosis of anorexia depends on the absence of menstruation and has theories which include fear of growing up, men and sex. There is very little information available in the literature which supports the notion of the pressure that society itself places on women. Instead this pathological framework sets out to 'cure' women with re-feeding programmes, and a system of reward and punishment for weight gain and loss. These serve to further disempower a woman by denying her of her basic rights, and may reduce her to the level of a spoilt and naughty child. Louise, who was being treated for an 'eating disorder' at the time, goes on to talk about the effects of her 'treatment' within a behavioural therapy unit: "On having every aspect of my life controlled I was left with no outlet to express myself. I felt totally oppressed and very angry at my oppressors. I witnessed one inmate being force-fed by the other inmates while the nurse watched on. As everybody had to stay at the table until all had finished, refusal meant that we all suffered. It felt like being a Jew having to push your friends into the gas chamber in order to save your own skin. The only other available target left to scream out my anger – was myself. I learnt to scream quietly. Self mutilation came easily to me. It was the only way to cope with and express my pain. There seemed to be no other avenue."

Strict 'treatment' regimes which allow limited outlets for self expression serve only to increase distress. The individual feels trapped into having to swallow what is being handed out without being offered the chance to express her underlying feelings. She is not being given any choices. Her reality, her needs are not being taken seriously. Other people have decided them for her; indeed, her carers sit and watch this "dietary rape" as Louise called it. It is not uncommon for a woman to have her outdoor clothes taken away and be forced to use bed pans rather than use the toilet. Yet the 1983 Mental Health Act code of practice states that people receiving behaviour modification should have 'reasonable privacy', should be 'comfortable' and should be able to contribute to their treatment plans. But no literature gives guidelines on how these should be practised. So units are left to determine and control a patient's care.

It is hard to have our needs taken seriously as women and be believed. We are not seen as being powerful; we are treated as 'victims', which is often how we see ourselves, so great is the persuasion – and often the covert and overt abuse we receive.

Most of us have thankfully taken on board the horrors of acts of rape committed against women and children. But our criminal justice system, for one example, still pays great attention to a woman's physical appearance, what she wears and was wearing at the time of rape, her ability to be able to articulate in detail the crimes inflicted on her. This of course adds to her sense of shame and further inflicts damage to her recovery. Many women fear coming forward in case they are not believed. While it may be the case that judges would be reluctant to sum up by saying to the jury as Judge David Wild did in 1982. "Women who say No do not always mean No. It is not just a question of saying No, it is a question of how she says it and makes it clear." He then went on to suggest that a woman only has to "keep her legs shut and she would not get it without force." Facts are hard to prove in acts of rape, especially when the court is made up of men, all looking for evidence.

Recently, 'Date Rape' has received massive attention by leading newspapers. Arguments broke out over the issue of consent, which caused much public debate. Innocence and guilt became issues of public concern. Generated by press coverage, male 'innocence' and the possibilities of female 'guilt' were highlighted extensively. Feminists were blamed for causing women to fear men and heated discussions about consent broke out. Despite individuals responding in anger to this issue (quite a few were men standing up in defence of women), soon it became obvious that this was really an issue of media power.

We are told that some women are 'dangerous' to men, but in reality, this kind of weighty publicity against women holds far more danger. We are led to believe that we have engendered our own fear of men. But it may not be the fear of individual men which frightens us, more it is a fear of male power in general. Our political, economic and cultural identity as a society is based on a hierarchy which is steeped in patriarchal and misogynistic beliefs. Our laws are made up by politicians who have the power to dictate laws which affect us. In this case a woman's right to anonymity in cases of rape was an issue, but, had anonymity been overturned, it would have prevented many women coming forward to report abuse.

Women have shouldered guilt in response to the rigid beliefs and laws about women's 'irrational' and 'provocative' behaviour since the Old Testament was written. It demands that we should feel guilty and powerless to change our situation and should expend our energies making changes to our physical bodies.

This leads us back to Naomi Wolf who talks about how women become exhausted through trying to absolve guilt through diets, electrolysis, surgery and many other expensive, energy using pursuits to find inner acceptance through seeking perfection in their bodies. 'This beauty myth is not about women at all, it is about men's institutions and institutional power. Self harm is about power and trying to restore order to the difficult and painful areas of our lives. It never succeeds in bringing much ease because we cannot 'control' our lives in order to feel peace within ourselves. It simply does not work.

Control arises from a system that believes in perfection and is dismissive of anything which does not fit into its rigidly held beliefs. Black or white, right or wrong, it organises and defines its own reality and calls everything else illusion. Our life's experience, our reality become lost in logic. We learn that to understand everything, to be rational and in control is superior and real, that anything else is 'false' or unnecessary and will bring chaos and disorder if not controlled; that our gut feelings are really 'false' perceptions of the 'real' truth. So we learn to deny and invalidate our own reality, or make it fit into society's perception of 'truth' and logic.

Anne Wilson Schaef talks about control in her book 'When Society becomes an Addict.' She writes: "We live in a system founded on the belief that it is possible to control ourselves, other people, other systems, other countries, even the universe. We spend much of our time, energy and money pursuing this illusion. We then spend equal amounts cleaning up the resulting mess. Our physical bodies suffer so much stress when we try to control our own feelings and emotions that it erupts in high blood pressure, ulcers, colitis, heart attacks and strokes. Our relationships with other people fail because we try to control everyone with whom we come in contact. Our planet is on the brink of disaster because of the elaborate and lethal defence system we have created in trying to control other nations."

The harm which we do to our world reflects the same harm which we do to ourselves. The weapons of war our countries produce to defend us against feared attack could metaphorically represent our own individual need for self protection. Our struggle for survival may feel like a continual process of self defence against known or unknown enemies who could strike any minute.

In this unstable economic climate, we may live in fear of losing our jobs or homes. This instability may cause levels of continued stress because we never know if or when this might happen. So we try to make the most of our lives by hanging onto whatever we can in the present. For instance, our relationships and homes are lavished with attention, but when the next bill comes in we react by getting angry with loved ones. We fear losing both our jobs and homes yet the very fear of loss may be enough to cause feelings which run so high that they engender family break up. It is hard to communicate difficult feelings to those whom we are close to. We may try to protect others from our fears because we do not wish to frighten them. But underlying this are our fears of loss and abandonment, the fear of being left and of finding ourselves alone without the ones who care for us. That place can feel vulnerable and extremely frightening. The greater our need to defend our vulnerabilities, the bigger the weapons we might use to protect ourselves. For example, some people may build up layers of fat to protect a fragile sense of identity, others defend their vulnerability through drink or drugs. Many of us hoard feelings rather than confront a situation which, although difficult, feels rather too risky to do anything about – until it eventually blows up in our face! While we might understand the risks, we would rather go on defending ourselves in the moment than worry about the future. Self harm is a way of coping in the present moment. So, for instance, telling someone that smoking might kill them is to miss the point entirely. Smoking is effective in blocking difficult feelings, especially anger. So to be deprived of a cigarette may cause feelings of anger which the person is unable to deal with in a constructive way. The intent in smoking, like any other form of self harm, is not to die but to get through the moment, the next hour and so on. So if life problems increase, so the feelings and the amount of cigarettes, food, drink, drugs used. Whatever coping mechanism has proven effective before will be used again, or maybe something different will be tried which might prove more effective. So someone might try other stronger drugs, yes, but it is unwise to judge their actions because we do not have the information which tells us why they need to defend themselves in this 'stronger' way. What has happened to make them feel so in need of self invisibility, because this is the effect of drugs? Drugs mask and deny important feelings, so deny human strength and potential. They make us feel invisible to ourselves. Rather like the anorexic who diminishes in size, who loses sight of her powerful self.

The illusion is that we can control our feelings, so we build these mechanisms to cope with 'dangerous' (enemy) feelings and lose our freedom in the battle of self rescue. I am not saying that educating people as to the effects isn't useful, I think it's very important to make sure someone understands the risks – but we also need to allow the individual some choice in this. It is equally as useful to ask oneself just who is being made to feel better when for instance the anorexic puts on weight, or our partner stops smoking because we have threatened them with leaving?

I will discuss this more later, but for now I'd like to move on to looking at some of the more disturbing issues of abuse and self harm.

It is only over the last 20 years or so that childhood sexual abuse has been exposed. Before that time it happened covertly, no one spoke its name or could believe it happened – except in some poor and violent families. Rape within marriage was also similarly treated. Now many are coming forward to report acts of abuse and people are left questioning their own formerly believed 'safe castles.' In short, this menace has struck home and has intruded into all of our lives and beliefs.

The idea of abuse is hard to live with. We can never be certain that abuse has not happened, nor will ever happen, to those we know and love. Although we might try and deny the idea of sexual abuse happening within our own families, just the idea of intrusion alone can build up an uncomfortable picture. Imagine being burgled, or maybe you already know how this leaves you feeling: confused and upset to have lost precious items but above all angry that someone could have broken in and disrespectfully touched or broken the sacred seal of your home. You are left feeling helpless to change what has happened but have to live with the knowledge that it did happen. Perhaps you want to redecorate and throw damaged goods away. While in time acute feelings change to become those of resignation, you can never quite forget just how the experience felt, and remain in fear of it happening again. Imagine now, being burgled every day or night and never being able to predict when it might happen, or be able to protect yourself. Imagine not being able to express how that sort of vulnerability feels?

Feelings of anger, fear, confusion, guilt and shame are all those experienced by the abused child. It is not so much the abuse that is so damaging, it is silence and confusing feelings which no one in the family acknowledges. Indeed it is the silence that binds everyone together in mutual shame. 'Hidden within the shame bound family system, abusive events are kept secret from outside the family, and are denied within the family as well' (Wise).

The perpetrator of abuse is often the last person you would expect to abuse. He is devious and abuses many times without this being obvious, sometimes even to other members of the family. He may be well respected amongst the community, be a parent, or be working in a caring capacity. Many trust his intentions, do not believe that he could possibly harm anyone. But within his show of outward kindness he operates in a silence which is lethal, causing his victims long term psychological damage.

Self injury is quite an obvious response to abuse. The need to "get rid of the filth" is often reported by survivors of abuse who cut themselves to get rid of internalised feelings of shame. Defending oneself against owning the abuse and surviving through transferring the pain onto the body – the effect of which blocks intense feelings of emotional pain that would otherwise feel unsurvivable. This is the symbolic language of self harm. "No words could describe how I feel" said one woman. "It is a way of expressing the unspeakable" said another. What words could describe feelings that go far beyond our understanding of them, but whose power urges their release through the most guttural forms of physical expression as in self injury? Yet many of us have been so traumatised by our early life experiences that other resources to express or verbalise our feelings are unavailable.

In my research, over 70 per cent of people who self injure report childhood sexual abuse. Some of those were physically maltreated, and most felt emotionally abused/neglected. Over 90 per cent of women I have spoken to felt unheard as children and were unable to communicate their feelings.

Self injury: self cutting; burning; skin gouging; hair removal and the ingesting of toxic substances, is directed towards self rescue and survival. Even if that survival means continuously finding oneself in a place of self violence – it is nevertheless better than succumbing to the internal pressure of feelings.

Research from the 1980's report links with physical and sexual abuse in children who have subsequently self injured. Wise (1989) describes how victim–survivors of abuse use coping strategies to survive a family system of abuse, shame and denial. The phrase victim–survivor, it is stated, refers to the person's physical and emotional survival of the childhood abuse, and the defensive abilities developed for ongoing survival. Feelings of victimisation are ongoing, especially so if the survivor has little access to actual memories themselves. If the abuse occurred when the child was pre verbal, prior to her developing the necessary intellectual constructs, she may experience feelings of annihilation without being able to link this to specific incidents. "It may be that the experience of annihilation, rather than a specific incidence of abuse, is being re–enacted." (Blessing 90). This may be why women say how difficult it is to describe their feelings and are unable to make links with the past. The past is simply too painful and not only that, the abuse was confusing for the child to place; she was unable to comprehend what was happening.

The persistent act of boundary invasion, the intrusive nature of abuse, is what is so damaging. And it is not so much the physical experience, more it is the persistent nature of having one's 'self' robbed without being able to verbalise the reality and thus deny ownership of responsibility. Abuse becomes internalised, but "it may not be that the survivor is reproducing actual abuses through self injury, it may be that she is trying to rid herself of the responsibility of its occurrence" (Blessing 90).

If abuse was not recognised at the time of it happening and the perpetrator(s) not held responsible, the child is left holding the shame and guilt. Later she may certainly feel that her body did all the betraying by allowing the abuse to happen. Her 'needy' emotions (which were not supported at the time) further 'betraying' her bid to forget those damaging experiences. Some survivors cannot remember details of abuse, but talk about feeling as if they do not belong to their bodies. The body is perceived to be separate from self and feels numb. Whenever strong feelings threaten to surface they are externalised through injury – there being little physical sensation on a feeling level at the time of injury. Many women say they feel intrinsically 'bad' and say they release their 'evilness' through self injury.

Shame and guilt surround both abuse and self harm. In talking about the shame bound family, Wise (89) cites Fossum and Mason (86) "Shame is often expressed covertly through attitudes of being over critical, self righteous, rigid, blaming, pleasing and placating." The need to control self and others may move into a phase where there is a need to release control and shame. Fossum and Mason list abuse of alcohol, drugs, food, sex, money, physical abuse, sexual abuse, verbal abuse, and self mutilation as routes of escape from excessive level of abusive control.

It is important to restate that sexual abuse may not be the one and only link with self harm. Not everyone who self injures has been sexually abused, but all the women I have worked with and have spoken to, talk about feeling invalidated in a world full of grown ups where no one talked about their feelings, where anger or violence may not have been physically obvious but lingered in the atmosphere. This sabotaged feelings of safety and often ended with an important parent figure leaving. So it could well be that the need for release and escape is reproduced through self harm. "An end to the suffering" was how one woman expressed her feelings. Survivors may re-experience this loss through their own physical bodies. Self blame seems to be part of this, "I thought it was my fault" said the same woman.

THE SECRET

You told me not to tell
And I never did.
I wouldn't betray your secret world.
You swallowed me whole,
Consumed my spirit,
What could I say?
There was nothing left to speak
I was there, available.
For you to love me I'd do anything
I sold you my soul Father
But the price was too high.
Now there is nothing here
Just a bloody wound which
Marks my passing

                                                Anon

SECTION TWO

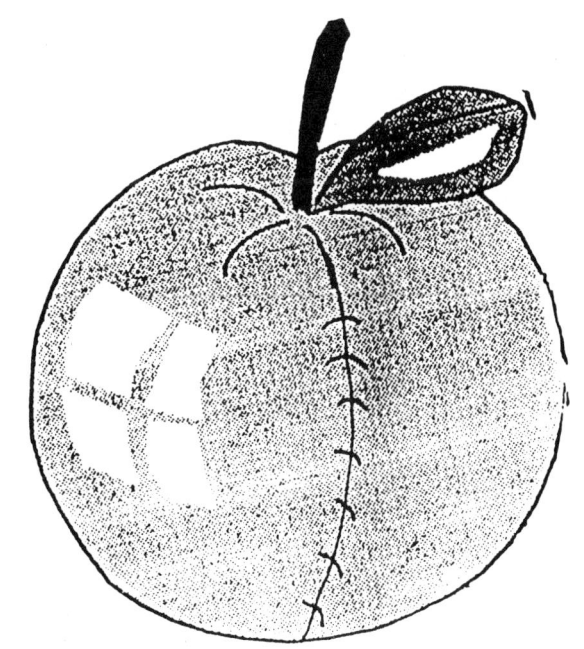

A FIGHT FOR SELF SURVIVAL - The body as a battleground

"My wounds are real. I can scream through cutting up my body. This is one thing in my life which is serious, nothing else is important – I guess I don't feel very important."Tina.

"If I was a man I'd have power. As a woman, cutting is the only power I've got."Beth.

"My body is the only battleground where I can do my fighting."Pat.

Self inflicted injury could be described as a radical response to feelings of total powerlessness and loss of self, a symbolic resistance to the power structures found within society which negate and silence women.

In a patriarchal society, laws have been used to attempt to describe a woman's 'reality', defining 'her' as the inherently weak 'other', subject to emotions of an unpredictable nature and a body with urges and passions which are 'unstable' or 'dangerous.' For centuries, the female body has been objectified, exploited and regulated by the control of the state, the church and the medical profession. In this way, a woman's experience and reality have been 'controlled', and her feelings and needs have been silenced and rendered less invisible.

Self harm could express the attempts women make at finding some resolve over power imbalances found in a society where rigid structures seek to organise and dictate what is 'normal'. We are told that it is 'normal' for a woman to pluck her eyebrows, or shave her bikini line. From these torturous procedures women seek to find acceptance – though need to continue these 'treatments' on an ongoing basis to remain feeling a modicum of self worth. Physical pain is part of the price, though after a time a woman's senses may become so conditioned to trauma that little is experienced on a feeling level. She simply switches off to the pain messages her body is sending. Her activities become an accepted part of life; she needs them to maintain her sense of being in the world.

Other women have their bodies pierced with holes for the wearing of jewellery. They also go through torturous procedures. But these, depending on which parts of her body have been pierced, and the rest of her appearance, will affect whether or not her activities are considered 'acceptable' to the rest of society. In Western society, body piercing tends to involve the young and the daring who often in general go against more widely held views and fashions of capitalist society. These young people are often vulnerable and may have little in the way of security or prospects. So they drop out of, or reject, the wishes of mainstream society which has miserably failed to notice their needs and look instead for a sense of belonging and visibility within their peer groups.

Like tattooing, face and body piercing may serve to express a person's individuality as different parts of the body are 'beautified' to suit each person. But having one's body continuously sore from piercing can become a way of living. The needed recognition and self worth aimed for, may fail to bring about the amount of satisfaction needed. As each of these fail, so more of the body may be adventurously and experimentally" beautified ". The risk of infection and even possible accidental injury is high but is anyway risked.

In their book 'Self Mutilation – Theory, Research and Treatment', B. Walsh and P. Rosen, discuss the many wide ranging forms of 'self mutilation' and "alteration of physical appearance and body configuration." They state that what differentiates self mutilation from other forms of 'beauty-enhancing' or 'symbolically meaningful' behaviours, is the 1) severity of damage and 2) the psychological state at the time of the self-altering act. So behaviours such as "simple ear piercing and the professional application of small tattoos" it is said are not considered self mutilative – because they entail less physical damage and psychologically the person is in a 'benign' state of wellbeing. They go on to say that these 'simple' acts are widely acceptable socially. But they say, "Self-alterations such as punk rock piercings and ritualistic scarrings among African and Polynesian clans entail more substantial damage. Nonetheless, since these behaviours are considered to be beauty enhancing or symbolically meaningful within a specific subculture, they are not considered truly self-mutilative."

So altering one's physical form in any way needs to be 'symbolically meaningful' or 'beauty enhancing' within a group or subculture if it is not to be considered a form of self inflicted injury. Anyone who alters their body in any way, in isolation and outside of what is acceptable, risks being psychiatrically labelled. Walsh and Rosen give an example of a woman who begins plucking her eyebrows as a beauty enhancement, but after a fight with her husband becomes fascinated with her eyes and eventually plucks out all her eyebrows and eyelashes. She is apparently then referred for psychiatric treatment.

Women who inflict injury to their bodies without obvious reason which might link their behaviour to a 'healthy' need for self beautification challenge all that is culturally and socially 'acceptable'. They strike at the heart of recognised female 'beauty' and behaviour. So the woman who plucked out all her lashes after a fight with her husband became the person in the partnership to visibly display all the marital hurts and was treated for her 'bizarre' behaviour. No reference is made to why they were fighting, nor is there any mention of the husband's behaviour towards his wife.

Women struggle to change how they feel about themselves through procedures such as liposuction which painfully suck away unwanted cellulite, or starve themselves on diets. Yet the idea of setting out to inflict damage on one's body is much more unacceptable as it is 'self' inflicted and appears more directly self violent. But women who injure themselves are trying to survive, just as women have battled to survive violence for centuries. There may be no visible conflict, no obvious perpetrator involved, but the causes of most of women's sufferings have been shrouded under veils of secrecy and silence and women have been blamed for causing or allowing their abusers to inflict damage on them. Women are left carrying internalised guilt, which builds up to dangerous levels. Without some form of release, it becomes explosive. Injuring one's body then, may serve to vent powerful and sometimes violent feelings which might otherwise build up to become more self destructive. Rather like releasing the valve in a pressure cooker, "Self injury lets off burning hot steam" explained one woman. When I ask the woman I work with how it might feel if they refrained from self injuring, the most usual response is that women begin to feel suicidal, or even contemplate suicide. The need to find a controlled release of overwhelmingly powerful feelings through injuring parts of one's body expresses the strength of women's ability to survive. The fact is that in the short term, anyway, self injury can be less dangerous than many semi starvation diets which can severely upset the metabolism, or can cause life threatening physical imbalances. Liposuction, apart from being agonising, can cause infection, damage to the capillaries, fluid loss, severe shock and even death – yet advertisements for diets or liposuction, disguised under campaigns to promote the 'body beautiful', are sold through attractive packaging. Setting out to inflict harm on oneself can never be called an attractive way of altering one's body form.

This poem was written by Anna, who speaks powerfully about the anger, pain and guilt she feels left with after years of having her body, mind and spirit "trampled" on. She expresses those feelings through her body.

Red as Raw is

Red as the ochre sun that threatens to boil cancerous skin.

Red as the iron soil that has been trampled by years of oppression.

Red as bloody sores.

Red as cancerous boils.

Red as skin that erupts like molten lava.

Red as healthy skin devoured by blackened dirt.

Red as cut skin, bloodied with amputated feelings that intermingle.

Red as guilt, fear.

Red as the blame that I am drenched in.

Red as anger that threatens destruction.

As women, the vehicles most readily available to us are our bodies. This may be the one area in our lives where we feel powerful enough to make changes.

While a man may make his mark in life outside of the home environment through work or social activities, a woman's mark may be made in her home and through her own body, marks made through childbirth, stretch marks through weight loss, right on through to self inflicted marks which defy all that is acceptable; we are either 'at home' inside our human flesh, or, most usually, are in some way disliking or hating what we see and feel about ourselves. As women our signatures and life stories are written on and through our bodies but we strive to keep this information hidden, or try to rewrite the reality – because the reality <u>has been at the source of our shame</u>.

In her book 'Shame and Guilt', Jane Middleton–Moz, talks about the power of guilt which has arisen from a shaming environment in childhood. The helpless child can do little to change the "constant attacks on their characters from the outside, or feel worthy when they are being treated as unlovable or unworthy." Shame therefore is the ultimate in helplessness and to survive that zero, annihilating position, the child repositions herself to make sense of the world. Guilt provides a reason: it is easier to blame oneself as a small child for what is going on than to blame others who are supposed to be caring for us. Guilt adds power and helps control situations which are confusing or beyond our control. As we grow up so we find ourselves constantly shifting into the position of self blame to become 'at fault' or 'the one who is really bad' whenever difficult experiences happen. And, we may find ourselves constantly trying to shift blame by sacrificing our own needs, perhaps by looking after other peoples, or working long hours in low paid jobs, or, maybe we try to make sense of our confusion through focusing our energies on to making bodily alterations.

But we have learnt to be ashamed of being female, for being a woman can feel 'dangerous'. Traditionally, the female body has been portrayed as dangerous, unhealthy, unstable and deviant. Aristotle stated: "Females are naturally libidinous, incite the males to copulation, and cry out during the act of coition." By positioning us as 'Other', we become diminished, objects for male gratification who can 'incite' men's sexual attention. Female circumcision, practised in over thirty countries, involving over twenty million females (Barry 79) involves the removal of most, or all of the external genitalia and for some unfortunate girls, the sewing up of the vagina to leave a small opening for the passing of urine or menstrual blood. A young girl's virginity then remains until her marriage. "It is not unknown for men to insist on their wives maintaining the stitches in their labia, in order to maintain a 'tight' vaginal opening, better for tight penetration and assurance of chastity" writes Jane Ussher (91). In some African societies the husband may open her vagina using a razor blade. "In one case, a husband poured acid on to his bride's vulva." (Favazza 87). (No wonder that women might cry out!) "But is it not a different representation of the same discourse that exhorts women to carry out vaginal exercises to ensure their man's pleasure, or encourages women to take hormone replacement therapy in middle age, in order to maintain a 'serviceable vagina?" writes Jane Ussher, in her book 'Women's Madness, Misogyny or Mental Illness."

The wounding and scarring of females through 'cultural' acts such as Chinese footbinding in which women are lamed for the 'pleasure' of gaining tiny, lotus shaped feet is an example of a misogynistic practice which ended in the nineteenth century. "The Chinese believed that being born a woman was payment for evils committed in a previous life. Footbinding was designed to spare a woman of another disastrous incarnation." (Dworkin 74). During childhood the feet would be bound tightly with bandages till bones were broken. This resulted in three inch stubs which were useless for walking, women needing to be carried or moving painfully about with sticks. When they attended social occasions or funerals the gathering were referred to as 'A forest of canes.' Men believed that a woman's small feet were erotic and that the practice had a "special bonus; namely, it caused layer after layer of folds to develop in the vagina, resulting in 'supernatural exaltation' during intercourse" (Favazza 87), Women were much confined to their bedrooms, not being able to move far and away from their husband's reaches. Ussher (91) likens Chinese footbinding to the restrictive practices of trussing Victorian women up in stays and corsets (often until they fainted), or the twentieth century women tottering on high heels in the name of fashion. "These women may claim to be merely exercising their right to wear the latest fashions; but they are not indoctrinated by the misogynistic discourse which decrees that women be both passive and vulnerable, not being able to move freely, which may mean not being able to think freely?" (Ussher 91). A woman's body like her mind become so straightjacketed by cultural conditioning that she feels guilty if she is not busy finding ways to 'get in shape'. Thus women become ashamed and frightened of their own bodies lest they are found 'too large' or in some way lacking.

An article has recently been written by Eileen Bradbury M.D. 'Aesthetic Plastic Surgery' which talks about women and plastic surgery. Women who see themselves as being large or misshapen are referred to the plastic surgeon looking for a resolution for their anxieties. "Surgeons and their patients are united in their understanding of the power of appearance in human interactions, and aesthetic plastic surgery is a profoundly psychological and social procedure." Women are seen for operations such as breast reduction, abdominoplasty (removal of abdominal fat) and liposuction and many of these women, it is stated, "have a history of eating disorders." These 'disorders' most commonly seen in the plastic surgery department are bulimia and compulsive eating. "The woman with a history of bulimia is likely to seek surgery to reduce her sense of being large." The article goes on to talk about the association between the need to control weight and size with the need to gain a general feeling of control over one's life – and also a concerning link with survivors of sexual abuse. "A major underlying problem which is often found to coexist with eating disorders is a history of sexual abuse." She goes on to give two examples:

"A 38 year old woman came seeking breast reduction. She had been sexually abused by her father when he was alive and had always tried to look asexual to defend herself. Now he was dead, she wanted to develop an independent sense of sexuality."

"A 45 year old woman wanted all her moles removed. She had been sexually abused by her brother and felt a sense of shame which manifested itself in these marks. She did not see moles on others, for they were not stigmatised. She also felt the need to punish herself by going through plastic surgery."

The article talks about women's profound sense of self shame which they project onto parts of their bodies which they find unacceptable and that this may lead them to avoid social situations. Another factor, the article states, which may cause women to seek surgery is familial and social estrangement. An example is given of a young Pakistani woman whose family had set up an arranged marriage abroad and had come to the attention of the surgeon for nose reduction. She had felt unaccepted and stigmatised by her family, her sisters had told her that she was ugly and would never marry, and was being sent abroad to marry a man much older than herself. The surgery was to help her escape this marriage and feel more accepted by her family. Unfortunately, the surgery did not work to her satisfaction and family matters were not resolved, and she ended up going through with the arranged marriage.

When a person in a group becomes stigmatised, is marked as the one who is different from the rest through their appearance, physical disabilities, temperament or whatever, then that person becomes the devalued member. The concept of stigma goes back to the Greeks who used bodily signs "designed to expose something unusual and bad about the moral status of the signifier" writes Goffman (63), "The signs were cut or burnt into the body and advertised that the bearer was a slave, a criminal, or a traitor – a blemished person, ritually polluted, to be avoided, especially in public places."

"Stigma is characterised by a pattern of social responses to particular groups of individuals. This includes those in wheelchairs, ethnic minorities, the psychiatric patient, and the disfigured. When these people are stigmatised, they are not treated as individuals but as stereotypes. The concept of stigma is one of devaluation, in that the individual who is stigmatised is devalued as a member of society... Stigma is an interactional process in that the power of the stigma lies in the acceptance of the stigma by the stigmatised. Because they are part of the same culture, they understand its meaning and may respond with a sense of shame and inferiority" (Bradbury 94).

So for an example, a woman who believes she is fat might avoid social situations for fear of peoples' reactions. People do stigmatise large women and she has probably heard many negative comments and inferences. Maybe also she has in some way drawn other people's attention to her size; through always talking ashamedly about weight; her endless desire to go on a 'strict' diet; putting up a front by laughing about her size to avoid feelings of shame. More stigmatisation arrives as she hides herself away from the world feeling more and more ashamed of her body.

Her generalised feelings of shame may focus on one 'offending' area of her body, such as her abdomen, which she strives to change through having surgery. Yet even if she succeeds to her satisfaction, she may well find that her self disgust simply refocuses itself into something else because her underlying feelings have not been addressed. She may then for instance, go on to develop bulimia and begin again to avoid social situations where food and drink might be an issue. And, other people may still define her as 'different' as stigmatisation allows for a person to become a scapegoat for other people's fears and anxieties.

Stigmatisation is rooted in shame, a need to hide one's 'offending' self away, or try to merge into society and reduce visibility. It can be extremely difficult for a woman to 'show' other people her pain through self inflicted wounds, for their reactions may be even more damaging. Since starting to write this book I have spoken or heard from over forty women who wish to share their experiences, not to mention all the many women I have known or worked with before. In all, at a rough estimate, I have spoken to over one hundred women of various ages from 16 years old to women in their fifties – ninety eight per cent have said that other people's reactions have been negative and even extremely damaging. The other two per cent are made up of women who have not shared their 'secret' with anyone else, or have only shared it with a caring partner, friend or counsellor with whom they have built a long term trusting relationship.

Women have shared their feelings of invisibility, which have, in part, been heightened by other people's reactions to their self injury. As one woman says:

"Once the 'normal' world sees my scars they won't accept them and on seeing them don't see me, only my scars."

Another woman, Julie, told me about how other people had responded to her:

"I have been upset. I feel very fragile after self-harming. I understand that friends etc. feel frustrated and puzzled, but they see the act, not what is going on underneath. I don't want them to ask me why I did it. I want them to ask me how I felt. The question 'why did you do it?' seems to demand an explanation of behaviour that shames me and also puzzles me, whereas 'how were you feeling?' might give me a chance to say what led to it all. It would be such a relief, so freeing, if somebody could say 'you must have been feeling so bad to do something like this', to recognise the feelings. I have occasionally been turned into a 'sideshow' for other people's love of the dramatic, or been so aware of the pain I have caused them, that guilt is added to my own feelings. I would be more than happy to talk to people that care about me if they feel hurt. It is a two way thing. But could I come first? Don't hijack my feelings."

One woman wrote and told me what happened when she showed a friend her wounds:

"I felt deeply humiliated by my friend's reaction. I've known her for ages and thought I'd have to tell her one day about what I did to myself. I took the chance and she looked at me like I had suddenly grown two heads, like I was suddenly different when I told her what my scars were really about. I know she was scared and worried about me but I am still the same person! It's been hard to cover up my wounds and say they were 'accidents'. It felt unreal, like I was lying to her and to myself. I was sure she didn't really believe me but I guess she believed what she could cope with. It's sad though; it feels like somewhere our relationship has changed and she has become wary of me, like I might be mad or something and I suppose I don't trust her like I thought I did. I feel vulnerable with her. I've exposed what was hurting me and it's been rejected. I'm not sure I'd want to tell anyone else I know. Please don't disclose my name"

The stigma attached to self injury follows women into casualty departments. While those involved in accidents are treated with respect and concern, a woman who has injured herself may find herself stigmatised by staff.

Sandra writes:

"I went into casualty having cut my arm. The Doctor asked if I was suicidal. When I said no, he asked me if I was going to do it again, to justify his time spent stitching me up. What does he know? I told him I KNOW where my arteries are! I couldn't talk to him after that and answer his questions so I went home. I feel awful because I can't stop cutting, like I am asking too much and should be able to cope but I can't. I give myself such a hard time then and cut myself deeper."

There are many other women who write in saying similar things and I will come back to their important experiences. Sadly and too often, women say how being dismissed by staff and carers has heightened their feelings of distress and isolation and this has increased self- blame and guilt. This has led to women trivialising and dismissing their injuries which have sometimes, in consequence, become infected. Or women have increased the damage to existing wounds by opening them up, or inflicting new and deeper wounds, thus in the long term raising the chances of severe physical, not to mention psychological damage. Typically women feel unheard and humiliated through having to justify their need for help, as if only a 'serious' (suicidal) intention is to be responded to while anything else is to be dismissed. The threat that help will be withdrawn if there is any likelihood of women returning to casualty leaves them feeling unheard and unworthy of support.

Even the labelling surrounding self harm minimises women's very real experiences. While injuring one's body can provide a means to survive, if a woman declares that she is NOT suicidal she may be seen as 'time wasting' or 'attention seeking'. Let us first take a look at some reports on suicide and self- harm to examine how 'seriously' each might be treated.

The terms 'failed', or 'attempted suicide' have been used to describe self- damaging acts to the body. Whilst some may be actual failed suicides, documentation before the fifties has tended to confuse self- harming acts with attempts at taking one's life – so any act which set out to harm became an 'attempt' at suicide. Since the eighties there has been a growing interest in distinguishing self -harm from attempted suicide and the term 'parasuicide' has been frequently used. But this term seems to describe something not quite real, a gesture at suicide. These 'gestures' have increased though, especially for women. Acts of self-harm described by Kreitman and Dyer (81) as 'non fatal self injuries', or the taking of substances in excess of what is prescribed, have, they say, "risen in frequency over the last 20 years" and is twenty to thirty times more common than suicide. Research which was conducted by Professor Colin Pritchard of Southampton University has established that there is a growing number of male suicides and a <u>falling number of female suicides</u>. MIND mental health statistics (94) report that:

"Suicide ranks in the top ten causes of death in most European countries, and is the second commonest cause of mortality in young men." And for young women, "They are particularly at risk of parasuicide: and represent 9 in 10 of all cases of non fatal acts of self–injury." Although exact figures are unavailable, at least 100,000 people are seen each year in casualty departments, say the Bristol Crisis Service for Women (a telephone help line and research project) and they say, at <u>least one million more may go unrecorded</u>. They also say that self injury is twice as common for women – so we can assume that these non fatal 'gestures' are saying something very real for women!

A woman who harms her body is seeking to find a 'serious' way to survive. Bonnie Burstow in her book 'Radical Feminist Therapy' includes an interesting chapter on 'Self Mutilation' and has outlined some of the purposes behind self-harm. While I will be addressing these issues throughout, I feel that listing them briefly would be useful. These purposes include:

1. A need to punish oneself.
2. To feel and see that one is real, human.
3. To bring back feelings from a state of numbness.
4. Attempt to end or destroy feelings.
5. As a form of communication.
6. To regain or feel some control.
7. A need to 'get back' at people.
8. As a form of resistance.
9. To get a 'high', a rush of energy.

I think that it is also necessary to say harming one's body may mean different things to different people, BUT may mean many different things to each person. Needs can change and can be more than one at any time. We are all changing individuals.

The many reasons behind the act of harm cannot be disregarded, or the 'seriousness' of the wounds, judged. Any underlying suicidal thoughts may be increased if a woman's actions are minimised and disregarded. Maybe the percentage of women who do go on to kill themselves would be less if women were taken more seriously. A woman's wounds speak the words that she cannot. Maybe the wounds are superficial, but then women's voices have been unheard and what they have said has been hidden and minimised. Perhaps the wounds she creates reflect her own needs to minimise what is real for her. Her reality is just too painful to face, to speak.

While the 19th century 'hysteric' became central to medical discourse, she was no more taken seriously than her twentieth century counterpart who cuts herself 'superficially'. Attention to the causes of a woman's 'nervous dis–ease' had been thought to focus on the womb which was believed to move around her body causing all manner of physical complaints. Madness became synonymous with womanhood, says Ussher and the 19th century marked a turning point in conceptualising women as 'mentally ill' or unstable. Though, writes Showalter, "During the decades between 1870 and 1910, middle class women were beginning to organise on behalf of higher education, entrance to the professions, and political rights." She goes on to say that simultaneously an increase of 'nervous' complaints such as anorexia, hysteria and neurasthenia had 'nerve' specialists trying to differentiate 'treatments' for different 'disorders' in her life. Women who fought to move away from their home confinement and work alongside men were opposed by the male establishments, and the guidelines for proper 'female behaviour' were reinforced. A woman's need for self improvement was dismissed and her struggle for self identity became the cause of her 'illness'. Thus, a woman's wholeness of being, her body and mind became separated and isolated from her. This enabled physicians to 'treat' and thereby 'control' women.

"It is clear, for instance, that many women fear to succeed in those spheres of activity traditionally assigned to men lest they thereby be disliked and regarded as 'unfeminine'." (Sayers 86)

I wanted to use a part of the piece that Louise wrote. Louise's reality became the subject of psychiatric pathology. Her distress and identity were broken down into various labels:

"I am a survivor of the psychiatric services. In the name of care and medicine I was locked up, drugged and subjected to ceremonial degradation. Some of the treatments I received caused greater problems that those identified as symptoms that commenced my psychiatric career. My entire life was reduced to a list of symptoms and ridiculed with labels that took away the meaning of my distress. Labels never alleviated my distress. I am a woman who discovered at an early age that a woman's worth is based upon her appearance; that the expressions of anger and assertion are not easily tolerated; that my place low in the pecking order has nothing to do with me as a person but more to do with maintaining an existing hierarchy of white male dominance. I discovered that for women and men the CONTROL of our feelings, perceptions and bodies was something that society valued, particularly for women: to be nice, neat and not too explosive emotionally was something to be admired. The oppression and discrimination that I became aware of were not only reflected within the mental health services, but actively reinforced, this by individuals who I was led to believe had better value systems and greater insight than I.

I learnt quickly that I was supposed to be a good and grateful patient; that 'insight' meant agreeing with my doctor; that I was supposed to be a helpless object that needed to be told what and who she should be. The acts of questioning perceptions or demanding one's rights became facets of the so-called illness. My world view and experience of living were unimportant. My distress was only acknowledged within a medical framework which is not my explanatory framework. My differences in perception have been dismissed as 'hallucinations'. The spiritual activity in my life has been written off as delusional'. My difficulties around eating were pronounced a 'disorder'. Whatever way I expressed my distress or dissent it was declared invalid, stupid or sick. It was drilled to the very core of me that I was incompetent and that my way of dealing with the official version of reality was invalid.

My whole experience was objectified, which I found dehumanising. I was never listened to. Each time I left hospital I felt like I spoke the wrong language or was on the wrong planet. My differences in perception are not hallucinations, but are real and have meaning. The disquiet I feel about injustices and oppression in the world is not stupid. In some cultures I would be seen as a gifted individual, but in Western culture my distress is medicalised in the exercise of social control, and also to provide a market for the pharmaceutical industry, who make big money out of people's distress. I do not view any particular expression of distress as pathological or intrinsically as a psychiatric phenomenon. I feel that people labelled as 'mentally ill' experience and express feelings the majority do not allow or open themselves to. To have expressed my distress in the way that it felt, could have at times resulted in annihilation. I had to hurt myself in order to keep myself quiet so I merely used the nearest target available – my body. I could not cope with the square hole that I was meant to fit. I was not a square peg. I tried hard to squeeze myself into it, accepting my prepared role as a woman, accepting global oppressions, and convincing myself that my new and different perceptions were not real. It didn't work. I became distressed denying what I felt.

I gave up ownership of my experiences. I had lost the right to self-determination. My self-respect was stolen from me. Ownership went to the blue file from the filing cabinet. Everything was categorised in pigeon-holes which prevented me from seeing how everything interacted. I do not necessarily experience the categorised distress in isolation. I don't have a 'Bulimia' day or 'Schizophrenic' day. This 'definition' and separation of the facets of my distress is not helpful. The rigid frameworks that psychiatry, psychology and therapy employ serve only to fragment and objectify people. They turn a break-up into a breakdown.

Society permits a narrow range of expression. When I started my tour of the mental health services I soon realised that the acceptable range was narrowed. I had to learn not to express anger and frustration towards what felt like torture. I started to self- harm during my first hospital admission, it was the only avenue I had to scream out my anger."

Phyllis Chesler, in her book 'Women and Madness' writes: "Given the custodial nature of asylums and the anti–female biases of most clinicians, women who seek 'help', women who have 'symptoms', are actually being punished for their conditioned and socially approved self–destructive behaviour." She goes on to say: "Men are generally allowed a greater range of 'acceptable' behaviours than are women. It can be argued that psychiatric hospitalisation or labelling relates to what society considers 'unacceptable' behaviour. Thus, since women are allowed fewer total behaviours and are more strictly confined to their role–sphere than are men, women, more than men, will commit more behaviours that are seen as 'ill' or 'unacceptable'."

Perhaps it would be good to look at other issues which affect women and see the scale of the problems being faced and brought to the attention of psychiatric practice. MIND studies show that more women than men are admitted to psychiatric hospital with 'obsessive–compulsive disorder' and 'phobic states'. One study estimated that 3.4per cent of men and 8 per cent of women are affected by phobias; 60 per cent of those who present at outpatient clinics have 'agoraphobia' and around 80 per cent of these are women. For depression it is estimated that 20 per cent of the population have depressive symptoms at any given point; the incidence is about twice as high in women as in men. Statistics on 'eating disorders' estimate that 60,000 – 200,000 of the population have problems around food and 20 per cent of women are likely to binge eat once a month, while 2–3 per cent are bulimia. Laxatives and vomiting are used by some 10 per cent of women and 1 in 500 women between the ages of 15 – 25 years require extensive treatment for anorexia. MIND information refers to research carried out by Dr. Andrew Hall at Leeds University who found that from 379 children surveyed, (average age 9 years 11 months) one in three nine year old girls worried about their weight and many dieted.

The conditioning of 'feminine' behaviour begins at an early age. Socialisation processes teach her to sabotage her own potential and to experience life through a much inhibited sense of being in the world. The nine year old girls mentioned have already learnt that to be accepted by their peers and the rest of society, they need to reduce their visibility and possible strength. In a few years time they may follow the struggles of their anorexic sisters who exist on the borders of survival, just.

Walter Mischel (66), a theorist and researcher in human behaviour, points out that children come to learn about the behaviour associated with their sex through observation rather than biological differences. So a girl observes the mother figure and learns from what she notices and hears. But says Ussher, the relationship between mother and daughter while being influential in the formation of the girl's self perception, is also ambivalent, because the mother has herself been subjected to oppressive conditioning learnt since her own childhood and prepares her daughter to fit into her circumscribed position. She learns "obedience to the social laws which define femininity; namely, deferring to others, anticipating and meeting the needs of others, as well as seeking self–definition through relationships" (Orbach 86). Yet far more women who are in relationships suffer from depression than those who are single. Women are failing to find the self fulfilment promised by glamorous messages about marriage and life long partnerships and become depressed. Yet in relationships men fare much better, and far more single, divorced and widowed men make up psychiatric statistics. The highest suicide rates for men aged between 15–44 have been found among those who are not, or are no longer married.

The relationships women are prepared for have been prescribed by and for the survival of male establishments. In relationships, women more than men will be the ones who carry any unease or 'dis–rest' within the partnership, which might result in emotional distress or 'disorder' and become defined as sick.

Particular groups of women may find themselves under psychiatric scrutiny single mothers, the working class, the poor and the unemployed, in fact, anyone who finds themselves positioned unfavourably within society, for vulnerability is not solely an issue pertaining to women. Men increasingly now find themselves at risk. Unemployment, for a start, has increased the despair felt amongst men who once had job security. In the last 10 years, the suicide rate amongst the under 25's has risen by 30 per cent. In 1990, nearly 600 young people killed themselves. As I said earlier, the largest majority of those were young men, who, research suggests, are four times more likely to attempt suicide. Gay and lesbian youth are also particularly at risk due to social stigma and associated isolation. Suicide rates are also particularly high among young Indian women.

Lack of prospects, hopelessness, social stigma, family conflicts and isolation are just some of the contributing factors which increase risks of emotional distress and in the extreme, attempted or actual suicide. Elizabeth Monk, of the University of London Institute for Child Health, did a random survey of young women aged between 15 and 20 found that one in five are depressed, one in five are found to be suffering from anxiety and depression and 10 per cent had contemplated suicide. But, social and economic factors aside, young people particularly are finding it difficult to communicate their distress and there is a lack of people to communicate to. So increasingly they slide into helplessness and despair which may for some spiral into taking drugs and onwards into crime. Males make up the highest numbers in prisons and psychiatric hospitals and are far more likely to be detained as 'mentally disordered offenders' than are women.

Young men are far more likely to blame boredom as a cause of distress, whereas young women talk about feeling depressed. Men are more likely to express their emotions through other people, for instance by blaming and becoming angry (and perhaps get locked up for doing so), while women are more likely to internalise their feelings, becoming depressed or anxious. Women use minor tranquillisers about twice as frequently as men do and may well try to lessen difficult feelings through prescribed drugs.

It seems that the way women and men describe themselves, how they act on their feelings, as well as how they are viewed by others will determine how and where they are 'treated': "Hospitalised women are in the majority in several traditional psychiatric diagnostic categories: psychotic depression, manic depression, psychoneurosis, and psychophysiological reactions," Breggin (93), or 'affective' and 'neurotic' conditions according to Busfield (86). Male 'diseases' tend to focus on pathological self indulgence such as alcoholism, drug addiction, drug induced psychosis and severe 'personality disorders' says Chesler. "Women's symptoms, on the other hand, express a harsh, self-critical, self depriving and often self destructive set of attitudes". Self blaming attitudes are more prevalent in women, whereas men are more likely to exhibit 'deviant', or 'other' blaming behaviour.

Let us look at some of the descriptions and attitudes surrounding self harm. The medical profession's terminology says that this is 'dysfunctional' or 'maladaptive' behaviour. But this limited view only takes into account what is obvious and understood by those who are, it must be said, in positions of power and judgement. The terms 'Personality Disorder' and 'Borderline' refer to people who cannot be classified as seriously 'mentally ill' but whose obvious distress challenges all that is understood as 'normality', such as in self harm.

Someone is deemed 'disordered' if their own perception of the world varies from the more widely accepted 'norm'. If they then express themselves in a way which challenges social order, 'act out', they may well be labelled, subjects of social and psychiatric concern. 'Personality disorder' labels have been filed on women who self harm. Unlike depression, which is seen as a 'female neurosis', harming one's body stands in brutal defiance of female 'passivity', the traits associated with 'femininity.' Whilst a sad and tearful woman may be tolerated, a woman who is overtly angry and frustrated is ignored. Women who are 'depressed' are tired and de-energised women; a woman who cuts herself seeks to find some energy, become 'high' rather than sink into submission.

Social learning theorists have said that girls are ignored or are chastised for assertive or aggressive behaviour. This same behaviour is accepted in boys and he is even rewarded by both peers and adults for his 'masculinity' (Sayers 86). Thus a woman who takes action through her body and injures herself is judged on behaviour which is associated with the male. Yet women who self injure have experienced the extremes of patriarchal interference in their lives and may have become so out of touch and separated from their bodies that they no longer feel real. Much of the shame and associated guilt which has never been expressed may have become so internalised that women blame themselves for having caused, or been vulnerable enough to allow, the abuse to happen. Women may fear their more 'masculine' power and assertiveness just as much as they fear their 'feminine' perceptiveness and compassion. Women who self injure are trying to take action and reclaim some strength in a world which has for centuries been disempowering and abusing women.

Anna wrote this descriptive poem about feelings which 'interfere' so much with her life that they 'burn' and 'scald' her.

<u>Feelings</u>

I don't want them
They get in the way
Always interfering
One minute I'm OK
Then they bubble up
Boiling – the steam rises
They spit, scald,
And I pull away – again
Sometimes I hate them
Even despise them
Get rid of them, take them away
Pleading – I shriek
They burn me once more
Run faster – I shout
Shouting louder
I block my ears
Shut my eyes
Scald my skin
In order to block out the pain
I don't want to...
...Feel them.

While doctors and psychiatrists are just beginning to accept that experiences in early life may lead to self harm, they are much more reluctant to believe that a woman's experience of oppression by way of being a female may lead her to injure herself. Even less likely are they to challenge their own practices which further oppress and 'fragment' women seeking help.

Sam, who was referred by her G.P. to a psychiatrist, for her 'self harming behaviour' found her life reduced to a set of labels. She complained of feeling patronised by 'experts', who she said, seemed to decide what was wrong with her and prescribed 'treatments' which further damaged rather than 'cured' her. On her first visit, she spent only twenty minutes with the psychiatrist before being prescribed anti-depressants and a further appointment one month away. When she subsequently turned up in Casualty after taking all her tablets at once, she was admitted to psychiatric hospital. On admission, she was searched for "damaging objects" and was confined to the ward for a period of forty eight hours. This she said, "Made me feel like I was an animal in a cage being watched, but in all that time noone really listened to me. They just wanted to make sure I didn't damage myself again, but what the hell good is that? Nothing really changes, except that now I am a 'disturbed' patient, with a diagnosis, a label, nothing worth bothering about."

Could this 'treatment' be any more enlightened than pre-nineteenth century practices of locking up 'the insane'? Ussher cites Alexander and Selesnick (67):

"Bedlam... was a favourite Sunday excursion spot for Londoners who came to stare at the madmen through the iron gates. Should they survive the filthy conditions, the abominable food, the isolation and darkness, and the brutality of their keepers, the patients of Bedlam were entitled to treatment – emetics, purgatives, bloodletting and various so-called harmless tortures provided by various paraphernalia."

While the physical environment which holds vulnerable human beings has changed and patients no longer have to sit on straw in their own filth, nor are they usually detained for long, there are still startling parallels to be drawn: Patients may be confined against their will, but instead of showing their distress, these days patients may struggle to sit on feelings, fearing to outwardly express their pain because it is no longer accepted and remains much more hidden from view. There are few 'safe places', not enough staff to listen and validate the painful reality of those who are being hospitalised: The holding chains that were, are visible now only by looking at the staring eyes, faces and shaking bodies of the unfortunates who are quietened with 'high tech' drugs; The 'tortures' have become 'treatments' such as ECT; Bullying tactics still happen by staff in the name of care and female patients especially may be subjected to emotional, physical and sexual harassment by patients and sometimes staff: The 'mad' who were once stared at by voyeurs, looking for Sunday entertainment, have become the daily fascinations of doctors, dedicated to finding a 'cure'.

In our new 'enlightened' age, diagnoses prescribed with liberal ease invalidate a person's subjective experiences but make them part of the 'symptoms' for 'Disorders' and psychological 'sickness'. As Louise talked about earlier, having her reality compartmentalised and isolating each part of her experience from the rest, she began to feel less of a whole person and became more and more fragmented.

Joanne, who had been sexually abused as a child, writes: "I've sometimes seen a psychiatrist, which I found to be a very pointless exercise. The only reason I've agreed, is to seem co–operative, and not have a section slammed on me. Apart from the usual belief of self harm being 'attention seeking', there are always those who will stick you into hospital, drug you up and treat you like an animal with no rights. This profession I find is the most ignorant of why self harm happens. I've had psychotherapy which failed, all of them desperately trying to find a 'box' they can fit me into, i.e. an 'alcoholic', 'depressive', 'hysterical'. They appear to get quite impatient when you don't fit into one." Joanne's experience of self harm and stigmatisation, plus her 'treatment' left her feeling: "condemned for what happened to me in my childhood, and reinforced the feeling that I am no good."

Julie has spent much of the last 12 years in psychiatric hospital: "Self harm has helped me survive over the last 12 years; without it I think I might have given up on life. I have been cutting since the age of 14. I believe it began due to the fact at this time I was very unhappy and was admitted to a child psychiatric unit. I found it very difficult to express my feelings verbally and was very emotionally upset and in need of a kind, caring, nurturing, supportive environment. Unfortunately for me, so called professionals were both physically and emotionally abusive towards me. In the end all my anguish and unhappiness was turned in on myself, due to the fact that people were not prepared to take time and listen to me. My only way of coping was by cutting, reverting into myself which brought more condemnation. Although it's been very difficult to allow hurtful comments, (such as 'you are stupid', 'look at the mess you've made') to sweep over me, they affect me, I cry, I feel anger towards them but am unable to show it and all emotions tend to be pent up inside. After all it's my body and if I could stop I would.

Now I am getting therapy and my therapist accepts me as a whole person and has helped me see that I split off when I am feeling tense and angry, hating of myself with total disgust and it's like I have to rid my body of something (?). It's like a cleansing process and it's like it is a necessity for me to see the blood and after a short period I am back to reality and very calm, like I'm a totally different person. Maybe in time I will stop needing this, I will feel real anyway."

If the medical professions continue to focus on blaming and trying to control the 'behaviour', so they will continue to overlook the symbolic attempts women make in trying to define what is real to each. By pathologizing her despair and by belittling or dismissing its true meaning, an important message is silenced and lost. A woman's feelings, like her body are reinforced as 'dangerous', in need of control. A woman who is accepted for being self negating, is just about tolerated if depressed (because there are 'treatments' for this) but is condemned if she expresses powerful feelings, or exhibits overtly 'self destructive behaviour'. So women themselves will remain fearful and intolerant or feelings — which might threaten the status quo.

PERSONALITY DISORDER

I don't want your labels
Your diagnosis, your pills,
I know what is wrong with me,
I'm not 'mad' or ill.
Just suffering from life's disorder,
In need of safety and support,
To work through all that's killing me,
In a place where that's allowed.
So put away your pens,
Throw aside the labels,
And just try listening to what I say!
I need to find control
Of the nightmares and pain
That keep destroying me slowly.
To go on like this, I'll soon be dead
So try writing 'understandably distressed' instead!

Anon

SECTION THREE

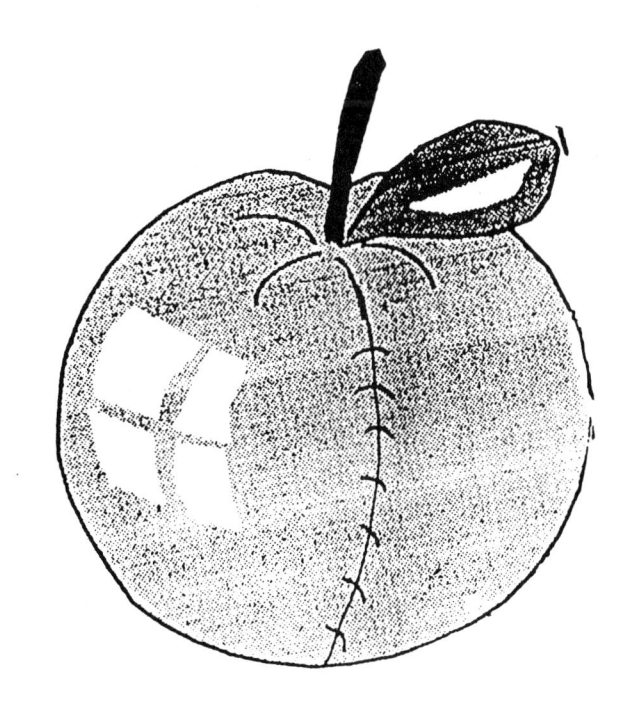

CREATING ORDER FROM CHAOS - A non verbal struggle for expression

Self harm brings some order to chaos. When there is little power in life to change outside circumstances, self harm brings some internal order. When there is no obvious reason to injure but the need is there anyway, it tells us that something, perhaps forgotten, in our lives needs immediate attention. Life is a process of learning to understand ourselves, self harm is a process in that understanding.

For some women who self injure there is a form of ritual in their preparations. In fact, the 'getting ready' can be an important part of the process. Sterilised strips, gauze, razors and disinfectant may be bought and stored ready for use. From what I understand, it seems that women who injure when they feel it is necessary and manage to prepare for this beforehand are likely to cut themselves less than if they delay or are in some way put off cutting. Scratches may be latticed across the arms, or are hidden on parts of the body. While there may be a great deal of blood loss, the wounds are more superficial than those inflicted when feeling intensely self harming.

Those who cut, through a build up of frustration and anger, who fear interference from others, or who are on alcohol/drugs, may create greater injury. Sharps found around the house, glass tin lids or other objects obtained from various sources are used but may inflict more severe injury. A sharp which turns out to be blunt can be more damaging than a new blade. More pressure is necessary and wounds made with old or blunt equipment can cause infection or severe bruising and tissue damage. Having a 'special' blade, or valuing equipment may reflect a modicum of self worth and concern over what one does and how it is done. It certainly gives women a sense of having some control over what they do to their bodies and when.

Judy writes, "It's like before self harm takes place there is an organised routine I have to go through. Making sure myself and my flat are clean and tidy and everything is in its place. I suppose it's a bit of an obsession but it's in control. I must say that cutting can occur very dramatically but usually it is planned."

Another woman, Ruth, says "Sometimes I used to delay it but then it sometimes took more to calm down or be enough, like waiting until you are over hungry or so full, you can't tell how full you are. Sometimes then the feeling that if you didn't carry on and do what you promised yourself, you'd be giving in to 'them' and being weak."

Some women keep knives and razors stored away, out of anyone else's notice. These hiding places give women a sense of having control over their life and body. But if others 'intrude' with her harming process, for instance, by disturbing, or trying to stop her, she may then go on to inflict greater damage than perhaps originally intended. Being 'discovered' has increased women's shameful feelings and has heightened guilt, and self hatred. Having others interfere with this 'private act', or her fearing that this could happen (because in the past someone more powerful has interfered or taken 'control'), so her need to defend her vulnerability is increased. In this case, women are less likely to worry about cleansing blades or wounds (which can lead to infection).

Joanne, who was sexually abused as a child, writes, "If I put off self harm, usually because my daughter is around, or someone is due to visit, I vent my anger on them, destroying many a friendship. I see them as objects in the way of feeling better. If this happens the self harm can change to feelings of suicide, hopelessness and that I am undeserving of friends. I can become so confused having not relieved the tension, I overdose."

The need to cut may rise in frequency as feelings of alienation, far from being alleviated through cutting, escalate. Women may cut themselves again and again and not feel 'rescued' by attempts to save themselves from overwhelming despair. Drugs or analgesics like paracetomol, even taken at dangerous level, may be used in an attempt at quelling emotional pain. Women learn how to 'control' drug dosage, not in an attempt at suicide but for 'time out' from their pain. As one woman said, "to prevent myself from dying from the pain of it, I take sleeping tablets to knock myself out." This need for 'controlled' space may last for a few hours, sometimes even for a day or two if feelings become suicidal. While the long term effects are self destructive and have a toll on the body, the moment is survived; the rest is put off until later. Julie told me about how her self harm began.

"It started when I was fifteen. My boyfriend left me and I went into the bathroom and cut my arm with a razor blade. The act of self harm was sparked off then, and always has been by intense feelings of rejection which leave me feeling depressed and isolated and hurt. My mother often tried to 'commit suicide' by putting plastic bags over her head, taking overdoses and once I saw her in the bath with a razor blade in her hand. The majority of these episodes were before my first self harming act and I think I learnt this behaviour from her. As a child I think I wanted someone to take care of me, feeling most of the time that I had to protect my mother from herself as well as from my father who was violent and drank a lot. My mother also drank a lot at times and my home life was very disturbed and insecure. I was not heard as a child, I cried by myself alone in bed every night, often frightened and having no one to help me. My mother couldn't help me because she was often frightened and hurt herself. My father didn't want to know and wasn't interested in me at all. My sisters and brothers were all much older than me and didn't seem to know what was going on. It was my secret and much too shameful to tell anyone. The powerful feelings I had such as anger could not be allowed out because of the damage that they might have done to myself and to my mother. I closed in on myself.

I cut myself now very infrequently, always when I'm drunk. I thought at one time that the drink produced the self harming behaviour, but think now that it gives me the courage to do it. A fairly typical experience is for me: I am rejected by somebody (always a man) and feel very hurt and angry. But I subdue the feelings. Instead I get on a kind of 'high' and get dressed up, go out and get drunk. I quite often start off in a 'good' mood and I am particularly lively. As I drink more and more the hurt feelings come to the surface and I feel unable to cope with the pain of them. I go home in a drunken (blurred) kind of state and decide to cut myself or take an overdose. I do it very quickly so that I don't have the time to think about it and change my mind. While I am cutting I experience a feeling of release and I cry a lot and the blood makes me feel that something is really wrong with me. I am not just imagining it all. I want to talk to somebody and sometimes ring people while I'm cutting, or afterwards. I want them to help me and feel that now I have a 'wound' I can ask for help. I sometimes get help, but not often. I go to bed and the next day when I wake up, I see the mess I have made and feel very weak, (physically and mentally), ashamed of myself and depressed. But also feel empty and almost calm, drained I suppose.

One particular time I cut myself and took an overdose, I got up the next day, had a bath, dressed my cuts and then wiped the blood off the furniture and the sick off the floor. The clearing up gave me a sense of control. It was my mess and clearing it up was also a way of clearing myself up. Later on that day I went shopping, cooked myself a good dinner and had a glass of wine (didn't feel the need to get drunk again) and tried to make plans for the future. It was as if I had reached a crisis or rock bottom point and after that I could only climb again.

This episode came soon after the death of my mother. It was as if I was saying "I can't take any more on my own, I can't take any more pain." And yet, ironically, I chose to express those feelings by inflicting more pain on myself. A couple of weeks later, I tried to throw a brick through my ex–partner's window, which was a deliberate choice between showing my anger or harming myself. I was very sorry the brick missed!"

Women who self harm are angry and feel isolated and condemned by a society who shuns and ignores 'unfeminine' angry women. With no outlet for anger, unchannelled feelings may begin to feel 'explosive'. This explosiveness may be defused through a variety of self harming acts. Bulimia, like self injury, may serve to purge the body of powerful feelings which cannot be dealt with in any other way. They are released through vomiting or got rid of through taking quantities of laxatives.

There have been moves in psychiatric research to link bulimia, anorexia and self injury into a 'deliberate self harm syndrome'. Literature suggests that there may be commonalities which connect each 'disorder' which make them part of the same 'syndrome'. Favazza (87), suggests that someone who self injures may also be bulimic and may use both 'behaviours', or will alternate between periods of each. Although women may certainly have problems both with eating and self harm, it is worrying that in the not too distant future, the many ways which women express their distress will be grouped together to form one overall 'syndrome'. And one pathology will describe a huge number of women for which one treatment will be designed and prescribed.

But focusing entirely on the actual self harm avoids dealing with the main issues, which then remain unvoiced. Similarly for women themselves, it is easy to think that the wounds are the only things in life with meaning – and attention is distracted from what is lost, that which has no place of belonging..

So, too, therapists can mistakenly become so panicked by a woman's injuries that they become blinded to the woman's emotional ' wounds' and only see the physical harm. Likewise, if I were to write this book on self inflicted injury alone, while this may have been important to a degree, I might easily pathologise the issue, which may bring further stigma to it. There is also a danger that I might stereotype the women who self harm and generalise. Rather, I feel it is better to enable some understanding of self harm within a context. While self inflicted injury is important, it is only important as one single issue which reflects many much larger and more frightening issues which are very real to us all. The attention self injury is beginning to draw now is only important in looking at why self harm has come about, why it is now important and frightening to so many. Just like the women who use this method of coping, it can distract attention from the underlying, more frightening difficulties which also need attention.

But self harm can also protect and allow women to survive and it is her choice to decide whether or not to explore the issue any further. It is her body, her control and having someone else take that away, not only disempowers her, it makes her method of survival invalid. We are all unique individuals and while this book attempts to highlight some of the issues involved, it cannot begin to describe the reality for each and every woman.

We have to keep in mind that coping mechanisms have been formed as a valuable part of coping with life's difficulties and that we all find ways to support personal survival. Self inflicted injury is at one end of a spectrum of a whole range of coping mechanisms – which we all use to some degree. Self injury enables some to regain a sense of having control over personal powerlessness. Quite a few professionals describe it as 'maladaptive behaviour'. I would argue that self harm is a necessary adaptation to impossible circumstances. Because we cannot get all we would ideally wish from life, we try to adapt our needs and cling on to what seems like the best choice in otherwise difficult circumstances.

People choose pursuits such as parachuting or bungee jumping to gain some excitement in life. In a national newspaper article, a fanatic of 'Base Jumping' (the practice of jumping from fixed objects at low heights) was interviewed. Apparently this 'sport' has a small following of about 600 people, who regularly risk their lives leaping from bridges or buildings in attempts to overcome fear through risk. The member being interviewed felt that if he sustained 'only' superficial scratches, the jump was considered unsuccessful. Having risked ones life was meaningless unless the body showed some 'evidence' of the fact.

This need for danger and the adrenalin rush which fear invokes can make the tediousness of life more livable. It can release tension and if injury happens, (and is survived) followers gain something to talk about. That it is followed mostly by men who otherwise live 'normal' lives, makes this sort of risk taking slightly more acceptable because there's little of the usual stigma of 'emotionality attached. Indeed, the interviewer went so far as to admire the daring involved and likened this to accepting the 'ultimate challenge'. Any broken bones or wounds would not be considered self inflicted in a case such as dangerous sport, rather they would be seen to be 'acceptable' and may even have some admirable value. But whilst this example may seem extreme, many of our 'accidents' if we closely examined them could tell a story. I wrote this piece for a woman in hospital once. It is called 'Joe Bloggs':

Joe Bloggs is in the cubicle next to the woman who self injured. While Joe is being treated with sympathy (he has a broken leg) the woman is blamed for having caused her injuries deliberately. The nurses are angry with the woman for her 'attention seeking behaviour' and inform her how time wasting it is to look after someone who may well be back next week with repeated injuries.

But much attention is given to Joe, who tells them in a hurt voice how he "Fell off the roof while fixing a tile." "Bloody ladder slipped" he said. Nobody asks further questions; it was an accident, a matter of bad circumstances, you know how it is. In reality, Joe was trying to escape from the unfinished row he had had with his wife and wanted a night out with his mates to cheer him up. He couldn't handle the situation, money was tight and his job boring. As he had told his mates often "She doesn't know what it's like." He was scared by the weight of his feelings, so escaped the unresolved issue.

Now Joe is in hospital on bed rest. His wife is at home feeling all this could have been prevented if she'd done more, handled the situation better. She looks at the housekeeping money and decides to cut back on food and take Joe in some goodies. He deserves cheering up.

His wife will continue to visit each day and will try to take Joe in something nice. The nurses understand his irritability at times, as life can be tough.

The woman is back at home, nobody understands her needs, even though she tried to communicate her distress as best she could. Her cries for help fell on ears who found it too hard to listen and know how best to help. She remains alone.

. . . .

Accidents can be the expressions of unresolved issues we haven't dealt with consciously. They can reflect our need to take time out, to physically and metaphorically 'have a break' and find space to think about what is really wrong and troubling us. Like the woman I know who said "The pain in my body reflects that of my mind", physical pain and injury caused through accidents can reflect what is going on in our lives emotionally. The larger the accident, the greater our need to find space for ourselves. Accidents can reflect a need for self-punishment. I know that when I was consciously trying to stop injuring myself, I had a series of minor accidents. It wasn't until I had started to like myself and really felt that I deserved far more from life than pain, that I stopped having accidents and illnesses. I used to get flu and colds every winter, even when I was self harming, but now these are rare. If I do get them, I know I need to stop and think about what they really mean to me, what I am needing.

We take quantities of analgesics to numb physical pain, but part of this need could be to alleviate guilt for needing time and some support. In killing the pain, we deaden the fear about having some space to just feel the hurts of life. I am not suggesting that giving up analgesia is best it can be very necessary but just give this some thought. All these various 'rescue remedies' we find on our shelves could be masking or denying what is wrong in our lives, what really needs our attention, the amount of love and support we have, or have not got for ourselves.

Some people find support and an escape from painful reality through Religion, to the point of fanaticism. Purging their 'sins' through self deprivation and self sacrifice, they forgo food and sleep for hours or days in their need for 'purification,' religious pilgrimages, lasting for several days, where pilgrims deny themselves of even the most basic rights of comfort. They are tortured from hunger, thirst, coldness, tiredness and physical injury from the long trek, sometimes undertaken barefoot. Yet followers feel 'delivered' from their sins, redeemed and cleansed from the 'evils' of the everyday world, more alive to life's meaning, they say. So should these culturally sanctioned forms of self harm and sacrifice be seen as beneficial, or as purifying to the body and senses of the believer, while self inflicted injury is condemned as purely destructive?

Commonly people believe self injury is painful, yet there is often an absence of pain, which is why most people find it hard to comprehend. Psychiatrists have been looking at the body's physical response to stress and have found high levels of endorphines, or natural opiates. These numb sites of trauma and also have the effect of numbing the emotions, so little is realised consciously.

During the war, many badly injured troops had little or no idea that they were wounded because physical pain was absent. Under stress, high levels of adrenalin and natural opiates allow the body to function in a state of high mental and physical arousal, but without the encumbrance of pain. Lowen (85) discusses the emotional defences of troops deployed in warfare. How, under the constant threat of death, fear and terror had to be suppressed, as did the horror witnessed on the killing fields. Just to continue in battle, the reality of fear and danger had to be denied. For to have experienced not just one's own feelings, but also those of one's opponent, may well have led to insanity. The whole experience of horror just could not have been tolerated and survived without suppressing and denying its impact. Men were therefore more able to operate without awareness of their emotional or physical state of wellbeing.

Some soldiers were unable to tolerate the stresses and found various ways of escape. Favazza (87) discusses self inflicted eye injuries and cites Cooper (1859) who talks about men putting stones, lime and corrosives in their eyes to cause infection that lead to Opthalmia. Apparently in 1809, three hundred soldiers became affected with this condition, though many were found hiding corrosives in their hospital beds. This same discovery was reported in 1945, says Favazza, amongst Indian troops serving under the British. Favazza cites Somerville–Large (47) who reports 375 cases of self inflicted eye injury among both British and Indian troops serving in India and the high incidence of eye injury among French workers in Germany who were trying to escape penal servitude. Somerset (45) reports on the low military rank of soldiers who had, by their own hands, sustained bilateral eye lesions during the first world war.

So we can begin to build up a picture of the lives of people who had little to lose by risking injury or blindness. Those who had little in the way of position, who had little choice, who could not tolerate the destruction and fear of annihilation – had nothing to lose by their actions. Also during World War One, some men were drawn to shoot or injure their legs or feet, or amputate their 'trigger finger' (so they couldn't shoot) in order to be discharged from duty. By emotionally or physically sacrificing a part of themselves, survival was more of a possibility. There was at least a sense of gaining some control over a potentially life threatening situation. Losing touch with feelings, risking blindness, losing limbs or fingers was unimportant: the need to survive was uppermost.

I am often asked whether women who injure are always aware of their actions, if they have a choice. On a few occasions, women say that they cannot remember injuring themselves, or have said they were not really aware of it happening. Although I cannot answer this fully, I have spoken to women who have no memories of cutting – who were also on psychiatric drugs which suppress emotions. These substances, which include neuroleptic drugs, can alter conscious awareness to the point where fear and physical pain are dulled. To 'escape' from this place and regain a sense of feeling, women injured themselves. These injuries, they told me, were deeper than on previous drug free occasions. And because there was no feeling to accompany the act – there was little to remember about it.

Women who feel alienated and dissociated from their bodies may have little recall of hurting themselves. For instance, one woman cut her genitals during a dissociative period and could not remember doing so. Over a period of ten years she had taken several overdoses but had never cut more than her arms. She had few memories of her childhood though had always been conscious of feeling numb from the waist down. Just previous to her injuring, she said she had experienced 'uncomfortable' and 'painful' feelings in her genitals and felt that this could be connected to her childhood. Several weeks later, through a series of flashbacks she remembered being abused by her father.

Those 'lost' memories can be experience as physical numbness but the body retains its own memories which may be triggered through a difficult present day crisis. The woman physically experienced a restimulation of abusive memories in her genitals. But because she felt that her body was now betraying her (by physically 'speaking' the truth) she felt her survival was threatened. Her numbness, a way of coping with the trauma, was endangered as her awakening consciousness brought sensation back to the area, and with it a surge of feelings which had until this time been suppressed. Also, by cutting the parts involved she had tried to destroy the 'evidence' of that involvement which had been too much for her to deal with. While in the process of reconnection with her 'lost' feelings and body senses, her self injury continued until she was more able and ready to assimilate the new information and deal with her feelings differently.

Survivors may disown violated parts of their body to the extent that it is as if they belong to someone else. The 'self' may become so split or fragmented it becomes multi dimensional, each part of the personality taking on its own identity to cope with the load. Multiple personalities within the 'self' may have a wide range of coping mechanisms and can attack each other if one threatens to expose the internal rules of silence (Blessing 90). The coping or host personality may have no recollection of how the injuries were inflicted and many not 'know' who did the attacking – so great is the dissociation.

Other women may not be aware of hurting themselves if punished for their actions or contracted by their therapists to stop. Because self injury can be such a necessary tool in survival, being put into a position where not only this lifeline is being severed but also support threatens to be withdrawn, may lead a woman to operate 'out of awareness'. She later 'discovers' herself badly injured, writes Burstow (92) who goes on to describe a case where the counsellor decided her self harming client was 'psychotic' and hospitalised her. The client continued to cut herself 'out of awareness'.

If a woman is pressurised into submitting to the decisions and needs of her counsellor, not only might she 'forget' having hurt herself but her injuries are likely to be more severe. Finding herself in a position of helplessness may engender an increase in the need to use the very behaviour she is supposed to be giving up. One woman I spoke to was contracted by her counsellor to stop cutting. The woman stopped cutting and instead set fire to her hand and ended up with first degree burns. This seems to show that while there may be an element of choice involved, there are a variety of different factors in operation, so the decision is not entirely free to make.

Not being able to remember why the need to injure oneself exists is reported by many women. But perhaps the subconscious mind has found a way to 'freeze' and forget that which was once too much to comprehend.

Again during the First World War, 'hysterical amnesia' was common amongst the troops. Men lost their identity for hours, weeks or months but continued in battle behaving rationally, writes Inglis (79). After recovery they had no memory of the 'fugue' period, as it was called then. This dissociative condition became known as 'shell shock' because it enabled physicians to classify sufferers as needing treatment, writes Inglis. It was also a more respectable label which implied that there was a 'valid' reason which caused men to lose their memory.

Since World War Two, documentation reports that amnesia, either the partial, temporary or the complete forgetting of an event, is characteristic of post traumatic stress, says Wylie. Recent studies on traumatic memory have explored the long term effects in survivors of childhood abuse. Briere (92) says that research has indicated that between 60 per cent and 64 per cent of clinical sexual abuse survivors sampled reported a loss of abusive specific memories at some point after their victimisation. A study was undertaken by Brier & Conte (1987) of approximately 500 sexual abuse survivors. Those who had previous amnesia and who were beginning to access some memory were quite often describing an earlier age for molestation and more sustained violence than those who had no known amnesia.

Yet dissociative states and memory loss are also reported by physically abused adults and those who have 'observed' trauma. Wylie gives an example of an ex–army nurse who forgot whole segments of her traumatic experiences as a nurse in Vietnam and did not retrieve these memories for 16 years.

But those who survived and returned from war, after some initial attention, had little in the way of organised support to help them adjust and integrate the experience into their lives. After the Vietnam war for example, there was no counselling support and few wished to hear what an impact war had had on young lives.

Often the emotions and true horror of the experience are lost, or are minimised or denied by survivors of trauma. It can be difficult anyway to express a painful experience, to find words and communicate the emotions which were 'missing' at the time – because they had to be suppressed. Many war survivors found adjusting to life too difficult and became physically ill or began to rely on drugs or alcohol to 'numb' their experience. Some managed to find some escape through psychiatry. Wylie talks about a study which was conducted in post war Britain which says that "15 per cent of all hospital psychiatric admissions were for psychotic amnesia." (The experience of war affected many lives). 'War Veterans,' as men came to be called, often suffered from depression, or became suicidal. Along with others, they found themselves psychiatrically labelled as suffering from a variety of 'dysfunctions' and 'disorders'.

'Post traumatic stress disorder' as it is now called, effects the lives of many. Liz Sayce, MIND's Policy Director, cites British research which suggests that about 50 per cent of women receiving psychiatric treatment and 20 per cent of men have been sexually abused as children. MIND also state the findings of a sociological survey conducted by Dr. Ronald Kessler, at Michigan University who suggests that post traumatic stress is one of the top mental health problems for women. The report says: "A lifetime prevalence of psychiatric disorder resulting from a traumatic experience was 12 per cent for women, double that of men. Among women, half the cases of post traumatic stress resulted from having been raped or sexually abused."

Flashbacks, or the reliving of parts of the experience are characteristics of post traumatic stress. Returning memories may be fragmented and whole chunks of time may remain missing, never to be recovered. The human brain cannot assimilate every image or experience as it occurs, even in normal situations. I know of women who say they have no visual memories of abuse: because they had their eyes closed at the time; it was too dark to see; they couldn't understand what was happening. A child may be too young to intellectually organise information, or the adult too frightened to be able to assimilate the experience. It is placed in a sort of limbo area in the mind and some of it, especially for the young, pre–verbal child, may never be accessed. Because there were no adult witnesses willing to acknowledge and verbalise reality at the time, so the adult survivor has little access to the truth.

> "It is not the trauma we suffer in childhood which makes us emotionally ill, but the inability to express that trauma so it is heard."
>
> Alice Miller

Burstow proposes that routine self injury may be suggestive of childhood battery or sexual abuse. Women who 'routinely self mutilate' "have been badly intruded on in childhood" (Burstow 92). She underlines how important this coping mechanism may have been to that hurt child's immediate and long term survival. But also important is that self injury doesn't become the symptom which defines sexual abuse. Survivors often talk to me about their concerns that they might have been abused yet cannot remember its occurrence. Not every individual has been sexually or physically abused, otherwise all survivors of abuse would self injure – which they certainly do not.

Whatever is true for each individual, it is true that self injury reflects the long term effects of feeling invalidated and of being unable to communicate difficult feelings. Or, of having one's needs disregarded by others who wish to feed their own needs for control.

> It's a silent scream,
> It's about trying to create order from chaos,
> It's a visual expression of extreme distress.
> Those of us who self injure
> Carry our emotional scars on our bodies.
>
> Maggie

Some women begin inflicting injury on themselves at an early age, others in their teens or even later on in adult life. Psychologists have questioned whether trauma experienced during pre-verbal years reflects an earlier onset of self injury. From my own work, I am not certain that focusing on when actual harming begins is necessarily very helpful. I know of women who have been through traumatic experiences in early

life but have not obviously harmed themselves until their teens.
Equally I know of women who begin injuring in early childhood. Physically manifesting distress through self injury may be ' obvious' signs which also need attention. Self injury very visually communicates distress, whereas a child without injuries who is unusually quiet might be hiding emotional wounds which go unseen. Equally a child who is noisy and disruptive may not have physical wounds but might be communicating her distress through her behaviour - which is ignored.

A child who is not listened to and whose value and importance in the world is abused or dismissed will feel unseen and unheard. She may come to believe that she is a devalued part of society. This child may go on to communicate through some form of emotional distress, or will manifest her disquiet through her physical body.

Teenagers or young people do ' copy' each other's behaviour and groups of youngsters may begin to self injure by carving patterns into their skin. While this might have a shock, horror value, it is important that onlookers understand that in today's climate, with little or no prospects for young people, they can feel powerless to change their situation. Injuring one's body can relieve the distress of boredom caused through hopelessness and can distract attention from what feels impossible to improve. Scars sustained from injuries can have value in that they make an individual feel 'different' from peers. Or, they can mark initiation and entry into a group. Carl Jung, in the book 'Man and his Symbols' (64) talks about the processes of initiation in tribal societies which were symbolic of the transition into adulthood. 'Novices' had to go through trials of strength in which he or she was fasted, tattooed or wounded, often having to endure both physical and emotional agony. Having a willingness to die was part of the process, which if survived, admitted the initiate into the 'higher' status of adulthood. In some tribal communities in Africa, scarification (a process of cutting and raising the skin to accentuate scar tissue) is used and even though now prohibited, this practice may indicate social status, or may be used to prevent disease.

For today's young people, there is little to welcome them into adulthood, it may seem like a place of hostility. Carving one's skin may serve as a psychological and physical test of endurance. Done within a group, it can initiate feelings of belonging. It may also serve to communicate a resistance to being 'swallowed up' and absorbed into the nothingness which may be lying in wait for some young people.

Self injury symbolises the process women go through to heal themselves psychologically, another test of endurance into and beyond the barriers of physical pain in order to ease intense psychological pressure. Scars may symbolise battles which have been fought and won, yet may also reflect the pointlessness of fighting that which is unknown. Alice writes:

"My world is very fragile and very shy and will hide away from me the second it feels threatened. It might be taken away, or worse, smashed to pieces. And then I really would be left with nothing. I protect my world and prove it to myself with my blood. I would like to be at peace with my world and to know it doesn't need such fierce protection. Maybe my own little world would still be there even if this battle wasn't going on. It would be living at peace with itself. I can exist without this fight going on and on. I won't disappear if the fighting stops. The fighting takes so much out of me. Maybe I've got to find a different way of fighting. I want to turn the light on and see my adversary face to face. I don't need to be frightened forever. But I want to see really what I am frightened of. It's just like Billy Bragg's song, I can't live with something I can't fight."

The visible injuries of self harm are less important than what the wounds are really communicating. I asked women what thought this might be:

Julie, "The first word that comes in mind is 'hurt' followed by the rage and wanting to be noticed, heard, to be loved, but feeling bad, unworthy and ugly, invisible to everyone, deserving to be punished, self hate."

Sheila, "Listen to me, nobody does, I want to live yet I don't know how to live another way. I'm also too frightened to die. I feel stupid, like I don't really exist."

Anne; "My self harm is probably as talkative as I am. It says amongst other things please hold me or touch me, then I'll know I am a real person. I want someone to hold me really tightly, my back against them and to be able to cry for as long as I need to, not for as long as they think I need to or for as long as they feel comfortable with. Living alone with no one to touch or hold legitimately, like a cat or dog, I sometimes wonder if I am alive or dead and have become a ghost. I watch couples cuddling, hugging in the street and it CUTS into me like a knife turning in my back and I feel I can't breathe.

It also says I'm so angry that my therapist wastes my expensive therapy time sometimes. It is like a power struggle I fantasise now and then of walking out and taking half if not all of my therapy fees.

I am also angry with my partner's endless promises and excuses regarding giving up smoking. 10 years now. Smoking and drinking are more socially acceptable addictions, mine is NOT. Mine does less harm' skin heals quickly, lungs and liver do not."

Nina: "If my self harm had words it would be expressing a multitude of emotions. The most clear feeling is one of wanting to feel my own body and pain after a period of disconnectedness. I feel this relates back to my experience of rape at the age of 4 by a distant family member. I learnt to cut off from painful and terrifying feelings. The cutting is also a symbolic expression of my deep desire to cut out my sexual parts which through overeating I have attempted to cover up and disown altogether. The day after cutting myself, especially when I'm with other people, I feel that the scars are something which no one can take away from me, they are almost precious to me - my own secret. I think this is an unconscious manifestation of the extent of sexual abuse which I told no-one about. It is also a very powerful anger I am only now starting to battle with myself when I feel the need to cut, by reasoning that it is more about wanting to hurt the person that did this to me, rather than myself, the 'victim'."

"The truth about our childhood is stored up in our body, although we can repress it, we can never alter it. Our intellect can be deceived, our feelings manipulated, our perceptions confused and our bodies tricked by medication. But someday the body will present its bill."

Alice Miller

SECTION FOUR

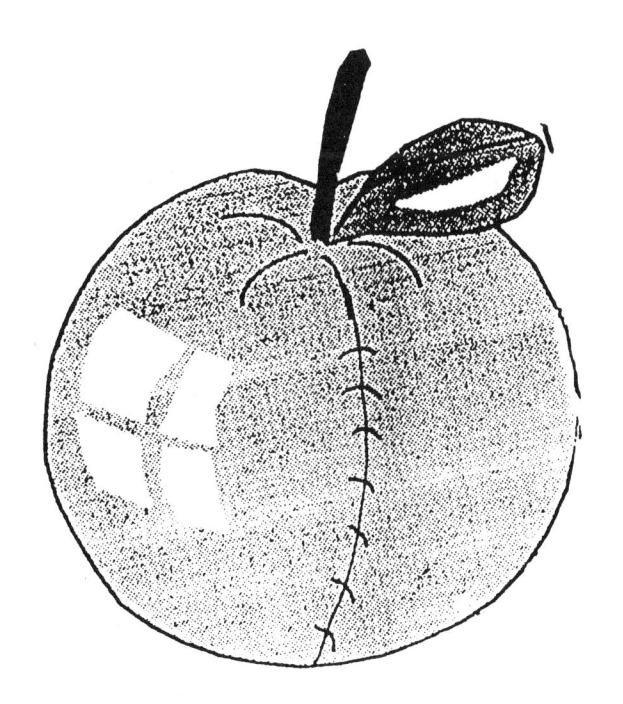

UNDERNEATH THE SKIN - The inner conflict

Maybe self inflicted injury is symbolic of how far we have collectively moved away from our true humanity. We have believed in solving conflict through violence and have sought to try and control things which do not fit into logical, 'man made' systems. Maybe it tells us that gaining understanding and greater compassion is very necessary if we are to halt our destruction and instead grow together as human beings. We are coming to the end of an extreme in the way we have dealt with matters. They do not work any more and we have got to learn a different way.

So can self injury be seen as 'irrational' when for centuries blood has been sacrificed through war? Yet world leaders have 'rationalised' the necessity of violence in bringing about peace. While many of us have realised that wars do not work, we still have wars and armed forces and enough nuclear defences in store to blow up the world many times over. We still live with a fear of being attacked and keep hold of weapons to 'defend' and 'protect' if necessary.

While self injury could be described as an explosive need to harm oneself, it is not in itself about being outwardly violent towards anyone else. Recently a panic response brought on largely through the media over the Beverley Allitt case has suggested that women who self injure might go on to hurt others. Yet there is no real evidence to suggest a possible link between harming oneself and injuring someone else. It is much more likely that women will blame themselves for what <u>others have done to them.</u>

To believe that people, more especially women, who in some way make visible their distress are therefore 'dangerous' to others, is a lethal track to follow. Women already feel guilty and this does no more than blame their methods of coping. It is a mentality which believes in what is seen at first glance and wishes to understand little else. That someone might become 'irrational' - because they have been subjected to another's 'irrationality' is understandable. That they will then go on to seek retribution through hurting another, overlooks the fact that self injury is about containing and reducing the effects of psychological damage. The need for revenge on another is essentially a male way of thinking and dealing with life's wrongdoings. Women already feel that they are wrong and this just heightens guilt. Harming one's body does little more than give some evidence of having sustained harm, when others are denying responsibility. I am not saying that women would never hurt anyone else, but the majority would never dream of doing so. Women are conditioned to target themselves first.

How can we blame people for trying to cope when there are so few resources to support survivors of abuse? Many cannot afford to pay therapy fees and resources that are free struggle with insufficient funding to enable their work to increase to match growing demand. There are many problems with using statutory resources, which is why many women keep a distance from them. Apart from the stigma of being a 'psychiatric patient' with few choices in your 'treatment', there is a problem with confidentiality. What a woman says or does can be passed on and discussed by others, recorded in her notes. If she discloses abuse, this can be reported, leaving her feeling guilty about having disclosed this information and fearful about what could happen.

Employers are unwilling to take on people with psychiatric histories. A woman who is known to harm herself can be sacked if found out, especially if she also works within the statutory services. Recent guidelines brought out by the Clothier report (a knee jerk response to the B. Allitt case) have done little more than list undesirable attributes for nurses. An 'eating disorder' such as anorexia can bar prospective nurses - as this is classified as evidence of 'personality disorder'. As an ex-nurse I cannot recall many nurses who could not be described as having some form of eating distress. Some were on endless diets, others ate compulsively. Eating or not eating were readily available ways of coping with a stressful job and sometimes we resorted to going down the pub after work if we'd had a particularly difficult shift and had patients die. But if nurses look towards counselling support and receive this long term, they also become an undesirable risk, so we hear from Clothier guidelines. Yet the stress of working with acutely ill patients alone is enough to warrant some regular support. All this does is drive women to further hide their distress, make it less visible to the authorities anyway. The idea that having human feelings which could be addressed through counselling might strengthen personal growth is entirely lacking. This is a negative and prurient approach which attempts to make women responsible for something which a patriarchal system does not wish to take on board. If a doctor or psychiatrist become depressed or suicidal, this might be seen as a 'symptom' of a stressful job. The job the cause; its effect depression. Few would wish to look for other added information. Yet women staff, doing traditionally female work, can have their lives scrutinised and any 'symptoms' of distress will be viewed with suspicion.

Regular, organised support is rarely available for either nursing or medical staff. All are expected to act 'professionally' - largely by keeping their feelings to themselves!

If strong feelings are denied or suppressed, they seem very frightening. When unreleased they can 'distress' our physical wellbeing and make us ill. But while the effects a of a build up of feeling (stress) are becoming better understood, all we are told by Department of Health guidelines is to avoid stressful or difficult situations Give up smoking, eat healthier foods and take more exercise. While these are useful, they teach us nothing about how to share and express our feelings in ways which are healthy and thus learn more about ourselves and how to deal with the world.

When I think about feelings, I think about the guiding aspects within all human beings from which we learn and grow in ourselves. In Western society we have learnt to fear our feelings and not to trust in our perceptions. So we try to control this aspect of ourselves by trying to suppress or deny its importance. Metaphorically speaking, we 'cut off' from the guiding aspects of ourselves and place our trust only in what can be seen or rationalised. Our lives become unbalanced and lose meaning as we look for ways of avoiding rather than working with how we feel. Yet the more we come to acknowledge our feelings, the more alive we become. In truth, there are no 'good' or 'bad' feelings: some just feel negative because they are painful of powerful and we get little support in dealing with them.

In her book 'The Living Wheel" (93), Annabelle Nelson discusses how emotional information is 'sensed' rather than is understood by the conscious, rational mind. Because this information cannot be processed in 'logical' sequence. we have used our 'rational' minds to undermine our unconscious, 'irrational' senses. Women often describe a 'sense' of being overwhelmed by powerful emotions and are unable to deal with them through usual conscious awareness. Injuring may then attempt to destroy this raw unknown which seems to fight for release.

The unknown areas of our minds are feared because we have learnt to mistrust our unconscious processes. Some theories have described how these less well known areas hold the keys to unlock great sources of knowledge and wisdom about ourselves. Our collective knowledge as human beings. Carl Jung believed that within each person's unconscious there lies a part that is connected to humanity unconscious as a whole, explains Nelson, the 'collective unconscious' as Jung described it. She goes on to say how Jung believed that within each person, lives a variety of archetypes. These archetypes dwell within the unconscious minds of the whole collective and are variously lived out by each one of us, for example, the fierce warrior, a primal strength within human beings; or perhaps the wise old woman who holds great sources of knowledge. If we lose touch with these aspects of ourselves, we lose touch with important information about humanity. These archetypes, explains Nelson, then basically operate out of control in one's own unconscious. So for instance, the warrior, instead of using her strength to overcome difficulties. becomes self destructive as that source of energy is suppressed. Likewise, in denying the wisdom of the old woman archetype, we fail to learn from our difficulties, become self destructive as that source of energy is suppressed.

Each one of us can affect and is affected by the rest of society. We are not separate individuals operating in isolation of each other, which is what we have come to believe. If we were to look at agoraphobia as an example, it could be that one woman's 'agoraphobia' is really woman's collective fear of our vulnerability and insecurity in the world. It is difficult to negotiate ourselves out there, even the street are unsafe for us to walk down alone. These collective fears then manifest in an individual, who begins to feel so unsafe and insecure she cannot begin to even venture outside. She is isolated and 'cut off' from the rest of humanity.

It is difficult to hold the possibility of a multitude of realities in mind if they cannot be logically analysed or be found to have physical evidence. We have been conditioned to use a scientific, dualistic model of thinking to prove reality and negate all other possibilities as being 'unreal' or false. So we are not supported for sensing or perceiving other dimensions. We might even be labelled as crazy if we did! If one explores the models of psychological theory, we can see how many theorists discuss the conscious and unconscious mind as if it began and ended with the individual, who is separate from the rest of society.

In the process of learning and moving on, I feel it would be useful to look at some of the thinking which has brought us to where we are today, and share with you some of the knowledge which has sometime painfully come to my attention, but nevertheless has come to affect thoughts and theory around women and our self harm. I feel I need to say that while it is useful and will I hope invite further thinking, I would warn readers that these next few pages may shortly incite some anger.

The conscious and unconscious mind was first discussed by psychoanalytic theory. The skin was said to represent the boundary of the self. Freud once described the skin as: "a special envelope or membrane resistant to stimuli." Lowen (85) describes it as "a protective shield" and says that the skin is representative of the surface consciousness. "The organism's perception of the interaction between inner and outer worlds." The consciousness, like the outer layer of the body, or the skin, is the boundary between oneself and the world outside - the self consciousness or ego, which enable us to organise ourselves within our environment so that we may exist as individuals. Theory explains that if the ego has been damaged during its development, a person may have little sense of self, limited, personal boundaries, and difficulty in distinguishing between what is inside and outside of her, or him self.

Lowen describes how the skin and surface tissues are sensitive to events in the inner and outer world. Thus, through our skin we are able to perceive and respond to external threats such as heat or pain which might otherwise cause extensive tissue damage. But if the skin layer is anaesthetised, such as through local anaesthetic, there is a loss of feeling and sensitivity. In effect, this reduces the consciousness in that area. Like sustaining local nerve damage, a deadening of sensation or feeling occurs. But the perception of trauma also involves the mind and its awareness. Lowen goes on to discuss how the surface of the brain involved in perception and ego ability to experience pain and react to it.

If the 'skin-self' has been traumatised, it becomes fragile without a structure to sustain a solid sense of being in the world. So a person may be unable to react to difficulties by removing themselves from them. Rather like holding one's hand over a flame and being burnt, they are unable to perceive external danger until it makes a painful impact. Thus, they may inadvertently be drawn into situations which further victimise, or may live in fear of being hurt but be unable to perceive whether the danger arises from an internal or external source. So perhaps through repeated self injury, not only scar tissue is increased but also the psychological boundaries between the inner and outer world.

But because the psychological barriers are insufficient to sustain feelings or events which arise, they may break down causing a flood of sensations. Lowen illustrates the idea of flooding by describing a river breaking its banks, obliterating the boundaries between land and water. Favazza describes this loss of self as 'depersonalisation': "Persons may retain a grip on reality yet feel that something strange is happening to their sense of self." Cutting may be a way to restore these self boundaries as it stimulates nerve endings in the skin and visually the sight of blood may allow the person to feel real or alive. In other words, regain some grip of internal order through focusing attention onto the outer limits of the body.

But while this is interesting, psychoanalytic ideas are impersonal, as if talking about an object or machine which has broken down and needs fixing. Instead of working with someone's diminished sense of self, in context to what has happened to them in their lives, they objectify someone by pathologizing their 'sickness'. For instance, the loss of self now makes up part of the diagnosis for 'borderline personality disorder'. Persons with this 'disorder' are described to be 'needy' and 'dependent' and have difficulty in forming relationships.

Firstly, this theory fails to acknowledge that women generally may have difficulty with boundaries. In giving and caring for others we are conditioned to have little sense of our own individuality and identity. Our 'neediness' has supported a male egotistic need for attention to his 'superiority'. A woman is not her own self, she walks beside or behind men, but not in front and has difficulty in recognising herself in her own right. She is flooded by the needs of others. But also and perhaps more importantly, a woman may have been abused, and using the term 'borderline' to describe women's experience not only denies what has happened to her, it supports the male need to retain superiority and power.

Favazza says: "Investigators consider most self-cutters diagnostically to be schizophrenic or borderline." He cites a number of studies (Pao 69; Grunebaum and Klerman 67; Burnham 69; Asch71) who, he says portray a 'typical' wrist slasher as "as attractive, intelligent, unmarried, young woman, who is either promiscuous or overtly afraid of sex, easily addicted and unable to relate to others. She slashes her wrists indiscriminately and repeatedly at the slightest provocation, but she does not commit suicide. She feels relief with the commission of her act." (Graff and Mallin 67)

Is it any wonder that this skin-self may become the target where any torments between the 'self' and the outer world are played out? Personally I do not know of any 'typical' wrist slashers! Investigations seem to focus on a woman's status, sex life and habits and show little interest in why she is distressed. Her feelings and actions are viewed as gestures, nothing too serious.

In trying to find some answers to women's self injury, Favazza goes on to illustrate his own perceptions by discussing a woman who had mutilated her body repeatedly. 'Janet', a client of his who had been cutting for 4 years, she said, because of her father's depression and suicidal threats. Cutting relieved her feelings of guilt, anxiety and 'episodes of depersonalisation' he writes. During her therapy, apparently, she disclosed that her father had given her 'special attention' as a child and it seems had covertly, if not overtly abused her in his convictions about 'their' mysterious and 'magical' need for each other. Favazza believed the "sexualized aspect of her love for her father, however, created enormous conflicts for Janet." He goes on to say how these aspects were '"central to her self mutilation." 'Janet' hated her female body and regarded her vagina as a "disgusting wound" and felt that life would have been better if she had been a boy. She detested her periods and sometimes cut herself to divert blood away from her vagina, we are told. Favazza, said he was surprised that in one session, Janet told him that her cuts "were like little vaginas and that she liked having her cuts sewn closed just as she would like to have her vagina sewn closed." Apparently she 'was particularly proud' of her stitches and kept her wounds clean, giving them huge measures of attention. Favazza interprets her "cuts as representing a vagina which were 'impregnated' with sutures, representing her father's sperm, the resulting scar tissue representing a baby. Thus her cuts had multiple symbolic meanings related to sexuality." But apart from Favazza's interpretations of Janet's cutting, maybe she was wanting her femininity 'sewn up' because she had been betrayed and left vulnerable by father's needs to own and possess her. Maybe in caring for her wounds and stitches, she was caring for her own lost childhood.

'Janet' had admitted her need to rid herself of the guilt and anxiety surrounding her father's suicidal behaviour. Perhaps also, she was extremely angry at her therapists interpretations of her life and his behaviour towards her.

It seems that before offering 'Janet' psychotherapy, Favazza had experimented with various behavioural approaches with Janet while she was under supervision in hospital. Apart from having staff watch her constantly, there were leather gloves to restrain her and tranquillisers available as necessary. Over a period of time, Favazza tried to get 'Janet' to fantasise a 'typical' cutting 'episode', and then if she began to cut, he would blow a whistle and shout stop! On one occasion she began to hyperventilate and the whistling failed to work, She seemed unaware of her surroundings. He says "Not even the glass of cold water which I poured on her head had any effect." Thankfully he abandoned his attempts at 'cure'! During their therapy sessions later, Favazza made up a 'no cutting' contract with 'Janet', which seemed to work in stopping her cutting, but at the time of writing it seems that she was on her way to developing anorexia.

While Favazza is at least honest about his non achievement here, he nevertheless battles on with his theories about sexual gratification through self injury.

In exclaiming the anguish self injury creates for patients, their families and therapists, Favazza expresses a need for 'an effective magic pill' or 'brief intervention technique.' After voicing his frustration, he goes on to say that a solid relationship over a long term is necessary for working with harming clients. But Favazza then suggests a 'pragmatic measure' (first described by Taylor 69) which can be useful for 'skilled therapists' in working with their clients. This measure, he says consists of challenging the self harming symptom to arouse an emotional response. Favazza cites Taylor, "Sexually challenging interpretations are especially effective;"for example, "I am afraid your skin cutting is a perverted form of masturbation." Favazza says that when the patient attacks the interpretation as untrue, the therapist responds with "The interpretation must be valid because otherwise you would not be so angry about it." The 'patient' it seems is put in an extremely difficult no win situation. For not only has the therapist fallen short of understanding, he is clearly using his own interpretations to overpower his client and thereby takes control. In effect, he has tried to dig under the client's skin to seek out something he wishes to find.

The minds of both client and therapist need taking into account surely? The conscious mind is selective, so Lowen tells us, it can focus on small areas of the external world and decrease awareness of the internal world. Objects and people can then reduced to images and this allows a person to manipulate others. According to legend, Narcissus, from which the term, narcissism developed, was a man who was punished by the gods because he has spurned his lover who then died of a broken heart. Narcissus was doomed to fall in love with his own image, which he did. He was so transfixed, he was unable to walk away from his own reflection and eventually died of starvation. In effect, he was drawn to see something which was merely a reflection of himself and was deprived of the food of emotional nourishment. He died still staring at something he couldn't move on from - an image.

But true to patriarchal ideas about women, Freud's concepts of female psychology marked narcissism as one of the leading feminine characteristics. And this became central to his theory of 'penis envy.' In examining the causes of women's 'neuroses', he argued that women were disadvantaged by their 'genital deficiency'. That to be born female was to be born a castrated, uncompleted male. To make up for this 'lack', women became obsessed with their own appearance. We have already explored how these male conceived ideas have worked towards supporting women's 'incapacitation' but Freud's theories didn't stop with narcissism. Millet (77) outlines how Freud believed that a 'passive' constitution, would be developed through "the abandonment of clitoral masturbation" and says Millet: "Freud hovers provocatively over such ideas as 'some secret relationship with masochism' and titillates us with reports of an appetite for pain."

Our supposed 'appetite' for pain has endorsed male violence and has significantly contributed to the way in which women relate to their bodies. It is hard to live inside one's own skin if what's inside lives under the threat of being taken over and hurt. Millet quotes Boneparte (53): "All forms of masochism are related, and in essence, more or less female, from the wish to be eaten by the father in the cannibalistic oral phase, through that of being whipped or beaten by him in the sadistic-anal stage, and of being castrated in the phallic stage, to the wish, in the adult feminine stage to be pierced."

As I have mentioned previously, women talk about being sewn up without anaesthetic.

Or, of being given insufficient local anaesthesia to quell the pain induced by these procedures. Women are 'pierced' with needles because of some belief that we will not feel it, or that it might do us good. We are so 'addicted' in our relationship with pain, why should a needle hurt as it plunges deep inside our flesh? Boneparte (53), in talking about both women and men's 'relationship' with pain, decides that men "repel the passive and masochistic" and are likely to be more assertive and aggressive, though are 'much softer' than women if undergoing surgical procedures. Boneparte seems obsessed with pain and piercing when discussing how women react to the same surgical procedures: "Women will suffer without flinching. These different reactions, at bottom, depend on the psycho-sexual response of their genital organs to the piercing, wounding penis." In other words, any pain inflicted on women is experienced sexually and reminds us of our 'desire' to be dominated and hurt.

Estella Welldon (92), decides that women express hostility and release anxiety through their whole bodies, rather than "through the one organ as it is with men." She discusses some of her own ideas around women and sexuality "women sometimes seem able to perceive their bodies in a whole way only when they are being penetrated during sexual intercourse." Welldon seems at odds with herself in trying to convince readers of her understanding. While on one hand she describes men's treatment of women, she nevertheless succumbs to her clinical judgments when she talks about "syndromes of self injury associated with biological and hormonal disorders affecting reproductive functioning." She then follows along similar lines to Bonaparte and discusses how women focus on their bodies and have a 'perverse libidinal gratification' through self inflicted pain.

Essentially a woman who refrains from sexual intercourse with a male, or who finds other substitutes, becomes a 'perversion'. These are the messages we hear through analytic discourse or anyone else who is unable to relate to women as autonomous beings. "Heterosexual intercourse is normal" we are told. so a woman's desires are only 'normal' if related to heterosexual lovemaking, which is then restricted to marriage and the making of children.

But according to theories and beliefs about women, we are dominated by hormones and sexual drives, all of which originally derived from men's fear and fascination about women, especially our life cycles. Shuttle and Redgrove (86) discuss how Freud had argued that women's vaginas were 'inferior' organs and that women experience very little in the way of sexual feeling through the clitoris compared to the penis. Both authors say that this was more to do with men's own feared loss of superiority, or his castration; "the bleeding vagina which might swallow a penis." Freud had argued that it was women who feared menstruation, yet the reality was more the other way around. Shuttle and Redgrove cite Faergeman, who suggests the idea of 'psychological castration', which say the authors " can mean anything form 'fear of love' to 'fear of loss of love'." "Faergeman believes, from his observations, that what the psychoanalaysts call 'castration' is a bloody bridge that leads from masculinity to femininity." Men's fear of finding themselves 'emasculated' and bleeding - like a menstruating woman.

Horror indeed for the unsuspecting male!

Ussher argues that men's fears and fantasies about women's menstruation were associated with witchcraft and powers that could render men impotent, cause famine and bring illnesses to many. Witches were thought to be responsible for the cannibalisation of babies.

The Goddess Lilith was named Adam's first wife and was also known as his other, 'dark' bride. Conway (94) writes that "tradition says that Lilith left Adam because he demanded full control of sexual positions." "Originally this Goddess ruled over pregnancy and sexual love with the owl as Her symbol. Patriarchy changed her into a demoness who preyed on pregnant women and newborns." Gray (94) says that Lilith was created Adam's equal and fled from Eden when her sexuality was denied.

Men's fear of and fascination for women have caused some to emulate the female genitalia, and even to attempt to destroy her 'malignant' maternal influence through self inflicted wounds. For instance, in New Guinea, men from the Wogeo tribe periodically incise their penises as a self purifying 'menstruation'. Favazza reports how some Australian aborigines are circumcised as part of the initiation process into manhood. Bettleheim (55) supported the idea of vagina envy, and that male initiation rites are used to assert men's ability to be equal with women. But some self mutilative practices are more clearly linked with men's fear of women's natural functions. For instance, in New Guinea, the practice of nasal mutilation is performed, writes Favassa, to rid males of 'contaminated' maternal blood, thought to have been swallowed at birth. "Wogeo men periodically 'menstruate', by gashing themselves when they are ill with a sickness blamed on female pollution." (Favazza)

Beliefs about women's 'dangerousness' and our abilities to castrate men have accumulated throughout history. The legendary Goddess Kali, was believed to be one such 'devouring demoness.' Kali, also known as 'the Dark Mother' represents both the creative and destructive qualities of life, death and rebirth. A rather dramatic image of Kali shows her squatting over her dead husband Shiva and devouring his penis with her vagina. Many took this literally says Conway (94) who describes how the priests of Cybele performed self castration in dedication to her. Apparently some worshippers offered the blood sacrifices of male animals. Today, Kali is depicted as a Black Goddess. Campbell (62) talks about "the terrible one of many names, whose stomach is a void and is forever giving birth to all things, a river of blood has been pouring continuously for millenniums."

But this 'devouring' aspect was not meant to be taken literally and has instead other more important means. "With Her vagina Kali takes the seed to be recreated within Her eternal womb." She also devours and destroys all life in order for it to be reformed, ready for another cycle of existence" says Conway. Kali's tantric worshippers realised that to truly understand and have wisdom, one must be willing to face all aspects of reality. Our negative limitations have to be ground down and destroyed before positive enlightenment and rebirth can happen. It has also been suggested that this 'Dark Mother' Goddess represents the dark phase of the moon. At the end of one cycle a period of rest and regeneration before the next begins. The cyclical forces of nature co-exist with women's own life cycles, her connectedness with nature and the universe itself. Gray (94) discusses how women's powerful sexuality and destructive energies experienced within the menstrual cycle became brought together in the image of a bloodlusting Goddess. "The welcoming Mother of death became perceived as evil, dealing in wanton destruction." Women's creative powers and sexuality were ignored in favour of the destructive potential of women. "The original image, of creative sexuality and death intertwined, has become horribly distorted."

Adam's temptation in Eden became Eve's 'curse'. Miranda Gray's excellent book 'Red Moon' tells us that the tree of knowledge represents women's fruitfulness (the womb tree). Eve picked the apple and shared this fruit of life with him and became cursed for bringing to humankind knowledge of the cycle of life and death. Christianity subsequently translated this into a punishment for bringing 'death to mankind': "In sorrow shall you bring forth children." Today, apart from experiencing physical pain associated with her reproductive cycles, a women's 'curse' is her sense of shame. She bleeds, she 'sins'. Women hide these feelings, cover their shame under discreet overgarments and take painkillers so that they may, for a while anyway, forget this 'curse'.

Women have talked to me about links between PMT and an increase in self injury. More than one woman has talked about her need to release some of the build up of physical and psychic energies associated with this time in the menstrual cycle. This 'time of the moon' or (lunar) month and its releasing powers are difficult to appreciate if women have consistently heard negative messages about their natural cycles and see their bleeding as a messy time of physical weakness and irritability. And if women fear their own power and perhaps have little feeling in their bodies anyway, any physical discomfort and 'tension' may be an uncomfortable reminder of physical, psychological and spiritual distress. These feelings are heightened at this time of the month because this is the time when women are most connected to our earth mother natures, the source of life and powerful creativity. Our life cycles are seen as women's 'mysteries' and women have been conditioned to fear what cannot be explained nor understood by the male.

But it hasn't always been this way. In some cultures the female body and her life cycles were celebrated. Rosalind Miles writes: "The birth of a new child out of the woman's body was intricately related to the birth of new crops out of the earth." In numerous other cultures, women withdrew into menstrual huts, ceased all relations with men and meditated during this time to renew the earth's fertility and allow the process of nature's energy to flow. With the release of blood, she allowed herself to surrender to the ancient Earth Mother in celebration of all life. Blood was thought to release great powers, much as the sacrificing of animal blood to the Gods was thought to purify and enrich the whole community. These animal representations of menstrual blood-sacrifice, says Shuttle and Redgrove, were held as sacred images or 'womb animals.' The pig is said to be symbolic of the womb and the moon, like the ebbing and flowing of the tide, the constant changing and transformation of life.

Sacrifice is the basis of primordial fertility rites, says Brinton Perera (81). She cites Eliade who points out "the fundamental idea is that life can only be born of another life which is sacrificed: the death by violence is creative in the sense that the sacrificed life becomes manifest ... at another level of existence. The sacrifice brings about a gigantic change." The victim is offered to the earth Goddess so that she might bestow good health and bounty upon the community.

The loss of blood is self inflicted injury, which may bring forth a renewal of energy if a general lowness or depression has been present. It could be an individual need to recover meaningful rites of growth and development which are largely disregarded in our society. But in the sense that self injury is linked with self punishment, this blood sacrifice could be symbolic of something very raw and fragile which has been lost and forgotten, a need to destroy the inner child self, a symbolic 'killing' of the neglected inner child's needs as they manifest - through the conscious, surface areas of the body. Not in the phallic interpretation of the raging 'Demon Goddess' image who seeks to satisfy sexual desire through blood sacrifice, but an attempt smother the raw needs of this lost child self, thus making her and them more immediately manageable.

Shirley talked to me a while ago about her inner child who she was so unable to relate to, she said 'it' every time I enquired about this aspect of her. Shirley's life story was brutal and harsh and she talked without feeling. She had needed to protect her survival so much as she grew up in various children's homes. She had had to displace her feelings and live without emotion. Now she couldn't connect to this part of her and wanted to push 'it' away.

Carl Jung once said: "Because there are innumerable things beyond the range of human understanding, we constantly use symbolic terms to represent concepts that we cannot define or fully comprehend."

Blood represents the life force and in self injury may be symbolic of the loss of connection with this inner life. The child with no home or parent to comfort has no place of belonging. So if and when a woman decides to stop injuring, these painful losses, which have not otherwise been dealt with, can surface alarmingly. But trust is an important issue here. It can be hard to trust oneself let alone allow anyone else, to hold this fragile child, allow her these needs and give her voice. That the right person will be there, who will offer support without wanting to take control, or "pull her out of it", is often too much of a risk for women to put themselves through. Little wonder when they have so often been let down by those who were supposed to be caring and supporting them.
Sally writes about her needs "I want to be held when I feel awful but I'm scared that I'll

be rejected or hurt yet again. I don't know how to love me and don't think I deserve to be loved."

Lyn says "It feels like I have never existed, no one really had time for me as a child, I sometimes feel suicidal now. A grown adult feeling like I need more than I am worthy of."

Julie: "Help me, love me, hug me. I was never heard as a child. I know that before I cut, I want to be held by a woman. After I cut I feel better like I want to cry a lot. Sometimes I do put off harming because I feel so angry that I don't know how deep I'll go. I feel that other people's responses are some part of why I cut too deep and do it so often. People call me attention seeking but no one wants to help me work out why I'm cutting."

Judy: "When cutting I feel total self hate and feel very vulnerable and like a child and would like to be physically held and comforted until I have come through it."

Patterns of harm cannot be changed through surface measures such as a change of behaviour; there needs to be a deeper but gentle exploration in finding peace and some purpose to life, a learning to mother and support the child as she grows and gains the love and self value that she rightfully deserves. This process can take a very long time. Even to begin exploring the survival structures that have kept a woman alive can feel like sacrificing her whole identity. To do this a woman needs to know that something better will enrich and will more than replace what is being given up, needing to trust and go beyond limiting coping mechanisms to develop a new sense of being and belonging in the world.

It can feel difficult to perceive this change, for when women have lived with the painful reality of life, and have had other people telling them to make changes, to explore better options, change can seem impossible. The truth is, life is very painful and may always be so, no matter what she does. And change can only happen if women are ready to move on. It really matters little what anyone else says. She needs to feel strong enough, or even desperate enough to think about something different. Women may not choose to go down this path. Or they may not be ready or trusting enough to face what is too difficult to experience. Choice is the issue here, women know what they need for themselves. Just as there are many different levels of reality, there is no one prescription for healing. Other choices and paths may be found which work. And these may also come to be changed as different needs are found and explored. Life is a process of learning. To face one's vulnerabilities and uncertainties, perhaps losing much in the process is no easy path to undertake. The road to what is called 'enlightenment' and healing is always there. But a bit like any path we might travel down in our physical worlds, the road might get too tough, we might want a break, or we change direction because the landscape doesn't inspire.

When I personally think about the journey towards healing, I think of the Goddess

Inanna who symbolises consciousness and transition. Inanna became sacrificed in the underworld for the earth's need for life and renewal. But her suffering was not about the relinquishment of sin, her paint was to remind humankind of the process of death, sacrifice, decay and rebirth - as part of the dynamism of life's Great Round, writes Brinton Perera. Inanna descended into the underworld and allowed herself to surrender to the process of conscious death but was reborn in a changed and much enlightened form.

Life is not static, we may be in psychological pain, sometimes unable to see its end. To sacrifice old patterns of behaviour can feel like a death of what we know, for we have clung onto them to sustain self identify. Giving them up, like the pain of sacrifice, to enter what is unknown, 'the underworld' or inner sanctuary of the Mother self. But as we begin to face our pain and fears, allow ourselves to go through the process of darkness, even though at times it can feel agonising, healing is possible. Though, writes Brinton Perera, "we will rarely approach such dismemberment if our pain is not already severe." During times of change, women may feel suicidal as a 'symbolic death' of familiar patterns is being worked through. Thoughts of 'escaping' through physical death may manifest, especially if these thoughts have always been an option lurking in the corner of the mind, available if needed, like an old and well known friend, or familiar enemy. What happens is that as we begin to challenge important parts of our lives, so these changes can shake up everything around us. The effects can spiral and extend beyond psychological changes to affect physical health and may alter our relationships with others. There may even be some temporary minor illnesses or unexpected difficulties which can cause feelings of 'being out of control'. These changes are normal and are a necessary part in growing and gaining self awareness, even though difficult to be with at the time.

We all find it difficult to accept something new in our lives when we are 'used' to going along with what we have, even though this in itself has been difficult. So, sometimes women seem to withdraw from this process and retreat into old patterns of harm. As feelings increase, so do the old and familiar ways we have of dealing with them. The worst thing that can happen at these times is that women are given, or give themselves, a hard time for their 'regressions'. It can make the situation much worse. Acceptance of the situation and an allowance for having these feelings and needs is essential. For as any pattern or way of being is being broken down, there may times when a retreat into the old and familiar is necessary.

Within this disintegration process, buried childhood traumas can surface and may result in feelings of disorientation or weakness. These may not solely have arrived from the individual's unconscious or past, but may also be linked to the 'collective unconscious' of humankind. Nelson (93) says "Deep feelings of unworthiness which may be based on the human race's karma will rear their head. Also, images from the ancient animal evolution of the Earth will come up. Jung talks about "The universal quality of the animal as a symbol of transcendence. These creatures, figuratively coming from the depths of the ancient earth mother, are symbolic denizens of the collective unconscious."

Women sometimes talk about seeing or sensing serpents, snakes or other animal creatures around them. Psychiatrists would see these as 'perceptual distortions' or delusional, symptoms of 'mental disorder '. Yet I believe these differences in perception are very real and have meaning. Jung talks about symbols of the unconscious, or messages of the mind manifesting through dreams or images. These perhaps crude animal like images, are in other cultures respected representations of spirit gods of life mysteries, projecting important messages to the observer. They are metaphors in our healing paths. Snakes can represent powerful magic, life changes. Conway (94) describes how the serpent or snake represents "Energy; beginning and ending; the Kundalini. " Nelson (93) refers to the concept of 'Kundalini energy' of Hindu origin: "a snake or a coiled serpent at the base of the spine. This is perceived to be "a creative energy of the spiritual body." Noble (93) refers to this as a "heat which heals and empowers, it belongs naturally to women through our biological processes." During menstruation, women shed a skin lining of the womb, much like the serpent sheds its skin constantly in the process of renewal: the holder of knowledge, inspiration and fertility. She goes on to say how Eve awoke to her womanhood through the serpent's bite. It brought forth her menstruation and creative powers, its 'sting' a knowledge of the process of life and a human connection with the greater awareness of the Earth Mother.

Since this time the image of the snake has had a phallic interpretation. Pictures of women lusting after snakes as if in desire for a three foot phallus, plunging and wounding. Again the belief about women and pain rears its ugly head! So, far from self harm being a need to create sexual gratification, cutting can symbolise a woman's need to re-own her own body and its needs and desires. The 'sting' of the snake may in this sense represent the poisonous messages we have received which have 'bitten' painfully deep. This also reflects women's collective need to regain what is rightfully ours, which has been stolen from us and polluted with fear and mistrust.

We all have the power to destroy. The problems lie in our fears of accepting that we do have powerful feelings and need to express them. Because we suppress or desire to control this energy it becomes destructive and explosive, uncontainable. So we try to get rid of it through taking physical action and strike at ourselves. My friend Louise once gave an analogy of monkeys being restrained in cages, then punished for their subsequent anger , via electric shocks. Initially, the monkeys tried to bite the surrounding cage but eventually started biting themselves in their fury. Taming these energies isn't the answer. We need to understand and work with this powerful 'primal' material.

Unfortunately, the incarceration and sometimes enforced 'treatment' is what often happens to women who harm themselves. This and other issues of treatment, therapy and support are the subjects for the closing sections of this book.

UNCOMFORTABLY NUMB

to dig the blade deep
into the arm and
twist hard

and yet feel nothing
as the spirit is purged

a symbolic expression
of an ancient hurt

in a place where
words are not
possible

the wish to alleviate
pain in a familiar
yet deadly way

primeval suffering is
temporarily anaesthetised

as the hunger for
destruction becomes
unbearable

and it is no longer possible
to disobey its commands

                Alex B.   (93)

SECTION FIVE

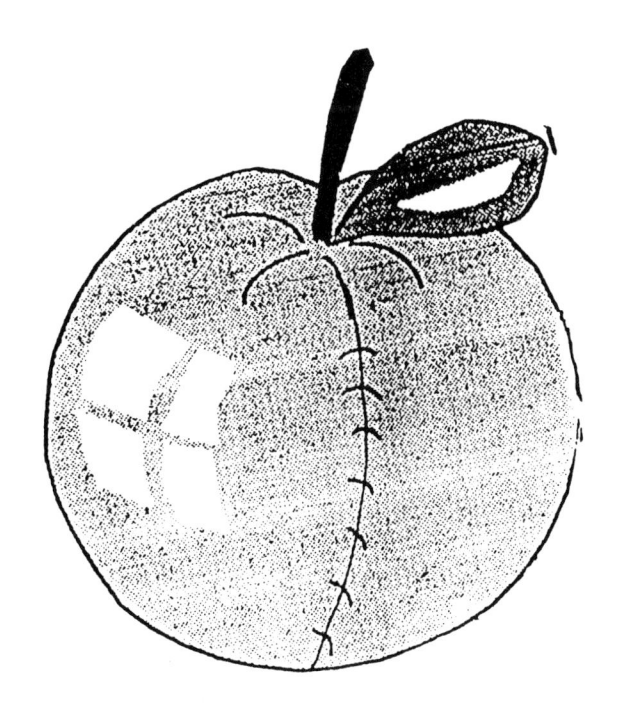

TREATMENT AND THERAPIES - Women's experience of help and support

Very often the 'treatments' given to women seem to do little more than find ways to enforce the containment of 'difficult' behaviour and women may find themselves incarcerated within institutions - with or without their consent. Far from being therapeutic, some 'curative' methods can even increase women's sense of isolation and perpetuate feelings of self blame.

Therapies found within the psychiatric system are often directed at making behavioural changes. The principal behind behavioural models are geared towards making changes in the way someone responds to life situations. Skinner (53) talks about the reinforcement of 'good' behaviour through response or reward. Behaviour deemed 'inappropriate' will "fade out of the client's repertoire by giving it little or no attention. " The following accounts are from women who have had this approach used on them.

Fiona said "My counsellor would only work with me if I refrained from harming but this was a huge pressure to be put under. I couldn't stop and I felt even more inadequate and guilty because I had to lie and pretend to be going along with it just to get help. I didn't want to be rejected, I've a lifetime of rejection."

This is what Ruth found : "When I was in hospital, the staff would only speak to me if I hadn't hurt myself. I was left to clean up my wounds and at one time they became horribly infected and my leg swelled up, I was in agony. I was asked to go and find staff to speak to if I needed to but they wouldn't listen to my feelings of needing to hurt myself; I just wasn't allowed to talk about what I wanted to do. I found another woman to talk to, a patient and used to talk to her, which was much better, though the staff didn't like it. They said we were colluding, which we weren't; it usually took the need away just being listened to and accepted."

Women have talked to me about how damaging this kind of 'treatment' is. A woman who self injures already has little self esteem, and to ignore and invalidate her way of survival merely reinforces guilt and may amplify any suicidal feelings which she may be harbouring under the surface. While it would be argued that behaviour modification therapies are not set up to punish, they are often experienced as a way of being blamed or made responsible for one's own pain.

McLoughlin (93) talks about the opening of a number of 'specified units' and the medicalization of self harm as an illness. She refers to an eight bedded young adults unit at the Bethlem Royal Hospital, who in their publicity state that "Patients may be informal or detained and we will consider most diagnostic groups, including personality disorders and problems of a self destructive nature (e.g self-mutilation and overdosing) . . " Interventions include: medication; specific behavioural and cognitive therapy; counselling for victims of sexual abuse. The emphasis seems to be on treating 'behavioural problems', pathologizing and detaining young people within a psychiatric setting for a period of up to six months - after an initial three week assessment.

Prisons and special hospitals have the highest incidence of self harm and much attention is put on 'maladaptive behaviour' and its reduction. A recent report on 'Self Injurious Behaviour In a Special Hospital' (Rampton) written by Duggan, Power and MacLeod, simply refers to traumatic childhood experiences as a possible origin of self harm. 'Patients' are described as having a 'low distress tolerance' and are 'vulnerable' female 'borderline', needing of close supervision. The report places emphasis on the need for practical problem solving as a way of developing skills to deal with distress on a day to day ward level and involving nursing staff. But Potier (93) has talked about women in Ashworth hospital and has highlighted staff's lack of tolerance to women who show 'too much subjective distress' - how assertive behaviour is punished while passivity is rewarded. She goes on to argue how the institutions are "by definition male establishments dominated by male power, where there is a seeming taboo on the appropriate expression of feeling." She expresses concern over the 're-enactment of abusive histories' through women being subjected to another's domination and total control over her life, the 'fear of reprisals' through punishment should she express anger. Potier argues that in this detached and cold environment, self harm may allow women to gain attention and regain some 'initiative' in the power game. One woman, Pat, expressed the powerlessness she had felt. As a young person who had been abused, she was placed in a remand home. "I was not powerful enough to be angry with them. Life held so few choices for me as a child and as a teenager. Now I feel so angry for taking responsibility for something that was not my fault. But it was a huge step to take."

Another woman, who was also abused as child and spent much of her life in various institutions, writes:

"I was sent to prison on remand. The magistrate said the reason why he was sending me to prison wasn't just because of the crime but because I cut myself so it was for own safety. I was very depressed and alone when I arrived and felt like harming myself. I had stitches in my arm at the prison. She asked me whether I felt suicidal. I said no but that I felt like harming myself, so I was told I would be housed on the hospital wing. I was searched by two officers. They saw the scars on my arms and gave me a disgusted look. The hospital wing was very depressing as you are locked in your cell nearly all day. The nurses never come to check on you so you could be up to anything. I was put on medication to help keep me calm. After a few days on the hospital wing I was moved to one of the main wings. This was a lot better as I was able to go to classes and mix with other inmates. I didn't feel like I had to be punished as I was able to get a cell of my own, which I preferred as I got embarrassed undressing in front of people because of my scars. Some of the inmates knew I cut myself and would call me hurtful names. In prison you have a lot of time on your own, so you think about things a lot. I would think about my past when I was sexually abused by my step-dad and when I lived in a children's home. I would get sad and feel like punishing myself and would look around my cell to see if there was anything I could use. If I couldn't find

anything I would get angry. A few times I told officers or nurses that I felt like harming myself, hoping that I would be able to
talk about why I felt like this, but their attitude was either "so what", or to threaten me with the strip cell. A strip cell is a cell without anything in it; some don't even have a window. When you are placed in a strip cell you are stripped and placed in a strip dress; this is a long dress which can't be burnt or ripped. Being in a strip cell makes you feel worse than before you went in. It's very degrading and you start to wonder why do people want to punish you all the time. You can be there for a few hours to a couple of days. Officers and nurses think just because you feel like punishing and hurting yourself you want to kill yourself.

It would amaze me because in some of the wings the cell windows were made of glass. I saw quite a few girls smash the windows just so they could get the glass to use on themselves. If there were groups to go to, about abuse, family relationships and rehabilitation, where you could talk about things, it might be better and fewer people would want/try to harm or kill themselves. I also think that officers should know how to handle someone who is feeling like hurting themselves instead of punishing them for feeling like that, or laughing at them. Prison did nothing for me; it made me resent the authorities . I think they could do a lot more to help people for when they get out .

Through studies in Ashworth Hospital; Liebling H and Chipchase H and Wetton (94) have conducted 'semi-structured' interviews with 40 women (representing two thirds of the current women patient population).
Reports into the background of women show that 60 per cent have been in care, 43 per cent in secure care and 85 per cent have received psychiatric hospitalisation. Most common early life problems were sexual abuse, family stress and physical, emotional and psychological abuse. Self harm had commonly
started in early teens, before institutionalisation, mostly taking place at home or in care. Overdosing accounted for 90 per cent of self harm followed by wrist cutting 83 per cent and attempted suicide 78 per cent. 65 per cent said they had intended to kill themselves at the time. 53 per cent said they self harmed more in special hospital than outside and experienced greater feelings of 'pressure' in being locked up with many rules and limited dignity. 90 per cent said they had harmed to relieve unbearable feelings. 70 per cent thought they had
greater problems than self harm. These were: being in a special hospital, fear of coping in the community, sexual abuse and alcohol problems. When asked how others responded to their self harm, 33 per cent said a doctor was called out and 60 per cent had their medication increased. 55 per cent were threatened with moving and restrictions, and 53 per cent reported being restrained.

Duggan, Power and MacLeod say that the incidence of self harm on hospital wards in Rampton has at some time or another involved most of the women. They feel concerned that nursing staff are being taken away from other duties to spend time supervising 'vulnerable patients', which can mean that "some individuals are seen to receive more attention than others; this in turn increases the likelihood of similar behaviour in others." Yet in the interviews conducted by Liebling, Chipchase and Wetton 75 per cent of women have stated that they would not self harm in response to watching others harming. Women may feel 'imprisoned' and isolated with their distress, desperate to find some relief. With no one seeming to be paying attention to their reality, some may well harm themselves because they have witnessed others doing so. Self harm may seem to allow momentary 'escape' from difficulties and can bring some needed attention to feelings of despair.

The Campaign For Women Within The Mental Health System, "questions the adequacy and effectiveness of therapies and practises within established mental health services which focus on treating symptoms in isolation from other issues affecting women's lives." They wish " to increase
knowledge and awareness of the lives and circumstances of women survivors of childhood sexual abuse who are within the mental health and learning disability systems and special hospitals because, too often, their expressions of anger have been labelled wrongly as ' challenging
behaviour' leading to self harm, alcohol and drug misuse, rejection and placement in the care system. Hospitalisation is too frequently a consequence of a history of such oppressive experiences for women." In a copy of a motion that went to, and was supported by NALGO Women's Conference 1992, TUC Women's Conference 1993, and NALGO Annual Conference 1993 there was concern that "women end up in special hospitals through criminal activity. It is then determined that these women can only be dealt with by mental health legislation rather than through the Criminal Justice System. While someone given a prison sentence will generally serve a determinate period in custody, under the Mental Health Act 1983 it is possible to detain people in special hospitals for an indefinite period. Once inside, the placement is degrading and humiliating, and the use of control by drugs is an accepted norm." And that "many of these women will have been sent to these hospitals as a result of self harm (often a response to sexual abuse), but that no attempt will then be made to address the causes." They also say that recent figures find the average stay for women in Broadmoor is nine years.

I have sometimes been accused of 'celebrating self harm`. While I do not celebrate self harm itself, I do celebrate women's resourcefulness in impossible situations. I truly believe that self injury reflects the dysfunctions of the larger structure and the more oppression there is, the more individuals will fight just to stay alive. Special hospitals are renowned for over-medicating women with tranquillisers, for the seclusion of distressed and angry women. These do little more than allow staff to 'restore order and control' while causing women problems of addiction not to mention the reenactment of her victimisation. Potier talks about excessive physical restraint by male staff, of the forceable stripping and seclusion of women who may have histories of childhood abuse.

Several women have talked to me about being abused, emotionally, sexually and physically whilst receiving 'treatment' in general psychiatric hospitals. Most have shared acute feelings of vulnerability and lack of safety within mixed wards. Also the 'abuse of power' through sectioning had they threatened to leave.

MIND has undertaken a 'Stress on Women Survey' looking at the services available to women in psychiatric hospitals. South West MIND, for example, sent questionnaires to nineteen NHS trusts asking them ten questions relating to sexual harassment and abuse policies, choice of women only wards and workers. Only eight responded though none could provide a copy of their policies on sexual harassment, despite being asked to do so. None of the nine trusts provided women only wards, apart from one who had a women only ward for the 'elderly mentally ill.' This lack of safety found one woman being cornered by male patients demanding sex. Another was attacked by a male patient. I have heard several accounts of harassment by male staff and one woman was even sexually molested on her way to hospital by a male car/ambulance driver.

What comes through time and time again in my work is women's fear of trusting other people enough to voice their needs and vulnerabilities. Little wonder if their fears of further abuse become realised by those in positions of power. I am constantly amazed at the infinite capacity women possess to go on enduring their pain when no one seems to understand.

"It's like being gagged and feeling that even if you could speak, no one would be able to understand you or would want to listen anyway. Maybe they wouldn't even think that what happened was important. I tell myself that what happened to me was nothing. I wasn't sexually abused. I don't really know what happened to me, suppose I was emotionally neglected. Nobody talked about their feelings and I was supposed to be quiet all the time, a good little girl. I rebelled as a teenager and upset my parents because I didn't want to do what was expected of me at school - pressure, all pressure to achieve and do well like my brothers. Now I feel like I need so much time to work it all out and feel guilty for wanting to demand more than I can have. I want a lot of space and time but I can't imagine what I'd do if I had it. I feel like a huge person tucked up tight in a little space and that's all I can have. If I were given this space, I imagine that I would explode my guts and I would go on forever spewing my insides out until I died. Cutting is like a controlled explosion. It keeps me alive but it's not enough because my needs are gradually destroying my body and I haven't much flesh now that isn't scarred. Hope you'll use this in your book, then I can say what it's like and share with others how hard it all is."

Kay

And how hard it is for women to allow themselves the right to be heard and to risk whether their pain will be taken seriously and supported. I think there is a huge danger of therapists and workers trying to fit someone into a particular category such as sexual abuse as a 'cause' of self harm. This can undermine and silence others who then feel less important. Kay, for example, told me that as a young girl, unlike her brothers who "always looked dirty and were fighting", she had been pressured to conform to stereotypical 'feminine behaviour' as well as achieving at school. She felt her wishes went unheard and that she had no outlets for her feelings, let alone to be the child she was, who wished to play and get dirty. Kay felt her blood expressed her rage and tears; it also "makes a bloody mess but it's less of a mess than my life."

Women find it so hard to think that they will be believed if they have no specific memories of trauma, and even if they have, it is a problematic area.

Nina said, "I recovered my memory of child abuse during therapy. I was astonished at what was coming out of my mouth. This was during a severe period of clinical depression and in retrospect it seems like the breakdown was necessary in order for me to uncover this buried, traumatic memory. However, since then, allowing myself to come to terms with this memory and accept it as mine has been made more difficult for me by extensive press coverage of 'False Memory Syndrome.' Now I feel torn between doubting my own memory, or accepting an unacceptable experience. Either way, I don't have much of a choice if I want to heal myself, so I am currently working on it with my therapist."

Jane wished at first to believe that her memories were 'only' a symptom of her 'illness.' "I didn't want to believe that my dad could have done this to me and caused me to end up as a psychiatric patient, a psychotic wreck. I wanted to believe that I'd had a happy childhood and it was me who was sick. False memory? Oh yes it would be easier to think I was ill and take drugs to quell the painful nightmares of my dad penetrating me. Luckily I see a therapist who believes me. She has never put the words into my mouth but has helped me incorporate my feelings and memories into my reality. Even though I often wish it were untrue because I 've lost my family now. They refused to go along with this and my Mum wants nothing to do with me."

Lucy: "When I started to remember my abuse I cut myself a lot more to try and stuff it all down again and forget it. Nobody believed me as a child so I forgot what happened to me until recently then I didn't want to believe myself, believe I had been a 'victim'. I felt bad and guilty about thinking such things about my parents and hurting them with these things."

The 'false memory' debate has been traumatic for women, especially in the early stages of memory recall. As memories return the adult has to acknowledge the hurt inner child's existence, her past victimisation and vulnerability, yet wanting badly to deny this new reality. McLoughlin (93) writes about "the blatant pathologizing of the said 'victim' . False Memory Syndrome positions the abuse survivor as ill: she is 'mad Jane', a witch or just a plain hysteric. This particular debate brings reminders of old Freudian analytic theory, his denial of the occurrence of sexual abuse within the family. Organisations such as the False Memory Syndrome Foundation, plus much media attention to women who now doubt their own memories, silence and discount many voices. Although no one doubts the reality of abuse, it seems it occurs in 'other' people's houses, never at home. Not possible. The family structure, no matter how it is perceived by those who had lived it, must remain closed to question.

McLoughlin cities an article in a USA magazine 'Body Memories' which questions why women coming forward with "symptoms associated with childhood trauma (anorexia/bulimia, post traumatic stress, fear of intimacy . .) are being called 'typical' experiences of women in the U.S." The article ends by asking why 'symptoms' of abuse are becoming 'normal' problems of women and questions what it is that needs protecting? One answer could be that it makes it much easier for many perpetrators if reality can be discredited in favour of women's fantasies? Another is that by 'normalising' women's distress, society does not have to take responsibility. And as I have already said, through medicalising women's 'symptoms' she can be more easily managed, while the real issues in wider society can remain 'safely' unacknowledged.

In a newspaper report, (1992 Guardian) MIND talked about the causes of women's distress being 'hidden' under their immediate difficulties, that "their distress is too often seen as a medical problem and social, economic and environmental factors can be ignored. Treatment on offer at the moment is frequently inappropriate or inadequate. Therapy, counselling and support to address hidden or root causes of distress is frequently not available."

Although Freudian beliefs once discounted abuse, there may be a danger that this issue may become something to seize upon, like a possession to be grabbed by those in power - such as in psychiatry. As I have said, abuse could become a possible answer to any number of 'symptoms' including self harm and can be 'treated' accordingly. Apart from anything else, this dismisses other possibilities and also discounts wider issues. Women become 'the problem' to be cured. Alice has written about what it felt like to be fitted into an 'abuse model'.

"Those of us who find ourselves in the psychiatric system get a hard time. We don't fit into the model which the system has worked out and has some way of dealing with. I don't know any specific incidents/situations I might be angry about. There isn't time in the NHS to find the causes and we are pushed towards the model of abuse - emotional or physical is seized upon. It is then attempted to be fitted into the abuse model and treated as such - a square peg in a round hole. Then the therapist and client both become frustrated because it doesn't seem to be working. And the client becomes resistant to being pushed towards the abuse model for fear of what she might be asked to 'confess' to try and fit into the model. She feels as if her therapist is missing the point; it doesn't feel like her situation which is being described to her. She feels more confused about really why she feels the need to damage herself and is less able to confront and explore why. Emotional abuse. What does that mean? Please find a different jargon for me. I don't fit into your jargon. I am Alice and the reasons why I self harm are as unique as Alice is. Please see and treat me as Alice and not a set of symptoms to be fitted into a model, to be fitted into a dot to dot treatment."

We need to get away from trying to work within a fixed framework of beliefs and instead explore what feels right for each woman.

Dusty Miller in her new book 'Women Who Hurt Themselves' (94) describes 'Trauma Reenactment Syndrome' (TRS), a broad term used for women who have histories of self harm stemming from childhood abuse. In this book she discusses her ideas about how trauma is reenacted by the woman through self harm, reenacting both the abuse and the lack of protection she received. But not all women fit into these broad descriptions and while some women's injuries may mirror the original abuse, not all necessarily follow this 'reenactment' theory, nor her ideas on what is useful. For example. Miller talks about the necessity of psychiatric hospitalisation for women giving up self harm: "A hospital staff is best equipped to protect the woman." No better options are explored for dealing with a crisis period than sending woman to patriarchal establishments. What is also worrying for any survivors reading this book are Miller's correlations between women who harm themselves and perpetrators of abuse." In exploring our attitudes toward women who hurt themselves, it may be useful to consider them as women who are inflicting abuse. Hurting oneself may be self abusive but this puts women down to the level of their abusers. Women then become 'dangerous', needing the same standards of containment and possible treatment one might view necessary for those who abuse other people.

Looking at the issue of being hospitalised while working through self harm, I have received a mixed response. Some have found it extremely unhelpful; others found having someone around for support has proven useful for a while. But all felt hospitalisation had been a last resort, which happened out of desperation rather than real choice.

One woman, Jude, said "I have received a lot of support over the years through the mental health system and until now it has been unsatisfactory. Professional attitudes towards me have been fear, shock and anger: "Oh, you do it for attention," "Stop feeling sorry for yourself." Instead of listening to me, I was briskly dealt with and left alone; no one wanted to know me as a person. I feel now I am receiving the help I have wanted/needed for the past 12 years. I see a therapist, whom I have been seeing for the past year. He accepts me as a person and is non judgemental - we communicate on an equal level. I feel very relaxed and actually feel I can see I am making progress although very slowly. As I write now I am on a psychiatric ward and have been here for the past month. This situation is not ideal and staff do not have sufficient time for me. I am here basically to have more talking time with my therapist who works on the ward and is able to give me more support if I'm here, rather than at home where I can only have one hour a week. At present we are working through a lot of past issues which I am finding pretty difficult and needing some extra support. I am very much isolated and friends are very few at the moment and are not very supportive. I really believe there should be more support out there for women like myself. Ideally I myself would like an alternative to the mental hospitals, as I myself do not see myself as mentally ill. A safe house would be ideal, somewhere one could go during a crisis where you would feel safe and people would be there for you and counselling was available."

During the time I have been writing this book. I have received a large response from women wanting to give information about their experiences of psychiatric support. Here are a few of these.

"I have had a mixed experience of reaction from professionals. The staff in the hospital day unit did not know I was cutting. The psychiatrist there did know but she used to sigh and shake her head and that was all. We never discussed it. The NHS psychologist that I saw was wonderful in accepting me and my feelings of wanting to cut and he patiently helped me to talk through how it felt before, during and afterwards. He never pushed me to talk about anything that I couldn't cope with and that was equally helpful."

Ann: "I see a psychotherapist who has been very helpful but when I admit to self harm he tells me it disgusts and makes him feel 'sick' in the stomach! When I challenge him when he says these things, I argue that he must have had many patients who self harm, he says he 'knows why I do it! He then says it affects him greatly! I can't win on that one. I see my therapist usually every two weeks and I 'promise' not to self harm but I burnt myself a lot with cigarettes when I was going through a very stressful time and he was away for 5 weeks. To me having to make a promise is not a very positive action."

Justine: "I suppose I am lucky and could afford to see a therapist privately. I had a 'dose' of psychiatry, hopeless, I had to wait weeks before I saw the psychiatrist after going to casualty in a very distressed state. When I saw 'him', it's usually a him, he referred me on to an NHS psychologist but I had months to wait. Again I saw a man who couldn't or wouldn't understand my self injury and overdosing. So I took over my own care and went to a private therapist who works with me as a whole person, not as a 'self harmer.' I much prefer working with a woman, I feel that she knows more what it's like from a woman's point of view and she doesn't judge me and my actions. We go through it together, like what is happening for me really matters to her. I've been seeing her for over a year now and it's taken all this time for me to begin working on my past. I needed to know that I could trust her not to reject me."

Nina: "It's about time we started talking openly about our experiences of being women. I am very conscious of this as my therapist is male, and even though he is very understanding, and actually openly expressed his distress when he first saw my burns. I know he can never know what it feels like to be penetrated against his will, and the long term ramifications of this."

Having a same sex therapist, or even to be given a choice in who women work with is extremely important. This might seem quite an obvious point but so often women are not given this choice when they look for support within the psychiatric system. That is, if they are given any help at all.

When women are referred on, they may not be given information about whom they might see and how this person works. Even after initial interview, women may still feel unclear as to length of time therapy might be offered for. And, fears are expressed over the possible withdrawal of support in the event of self harm occurring. There seems to be a basic lack of information about what therapy can and cannot offer women whilst going through periods of emotional crises and thereafter. This state of unknowingness can be very frightening and to survivors of abuse it may cause additional feelings of powerlessness and add to emotional blocks around trust and vulnerability. Women wonder whether therapists can be trusted to be with them in times of crisis, and if they are really able to listen to the depth of raw pain which may be seen which may be seen manifesting through self inflicted harm.

Any support offered through the NHS seems to vary from region to region throughout the country. And because resources are so few, whether someone gets support, and what this might be, may rely on a woman being able to articulate her needs. Sometimes it could even be put down to luck. A couple of women I have spoken to have had support from their G.P's; others have no support whatsoever. A couple of women have been given support at a day hospital where they have received regular individual counselling and have key workers - this is a rare exception. Others using day hospitals have had to rely on asking different members of staff who might be 'spared' to sit and listen. In some units there are too few staff to go round and women feel unseen and unheard amongst other more 'disturbed' patients. While a number of women have been referred to NHS psychologists, several have reported the work coming to an abrupt end because the therapist has left. Women have felt abandoned, perhaps unclear as to whether they will be further referred, unsure if they want to go through the process of building up trust with anyone else.

One woman had been asking for help over some months without success. During this time she had become very distressed and her self harm had escalated to the point where she was admitted to hospital with quite a severe injury. After discharge, and with the backing of a relative (who is a psychologist), she was given therapy from a psychologist and support from a community psychiatric nurse and a psychiatrist. Previously, while she knew she wanted help, she didn't know what might be useful to her or how to go about getting it. "At last I was being taken seriously. But it took all that to find out about what was on offer and to be given something useful. You need someone to help you get through the maze and to push for something to happen. Now I have good support and they listen seriously to what I am saying."

Some people have found support from their community mental health teams. The Bristol Crisis Service for Women says that although the availability of support varies from one area to another, women being referred to psychologists, psychotherapists, psychiatrists or CPN's, through a hospital or Community Mental Health Team, need to check what is on offer - that counselling time and space to talk can be given. And I wish to add, for a woman to take control of what happens to her, it is necessary for her to have some assurance that any support will be offered regularly over a period of time, for as long as she feels she needs.

I personally work from a person centred and feminist perspective in support groups and in any individual counselling work. I feel it is very necessary and empowering for women to feel that they are in charge of what happens during sessions. Usually when women make contact, they have arrived at the point where self harm is becoming very problematic to them, though sometimes they have been pressurised by social workers, G.P's, or others who out of desperation have put women in touch. But sorting through a woman's readiness for challenging self harm can be made more complicated by other people's worries about her alarming behaviour. Yet these same people would not think of intervening with a woman was in an abusive relationship for example. Burstow (92) writes " I know of no counsellors who would forcibly stop women from continuing these courses." As with any painful relationship, a woman may not yet be ready to leave her self harm behind. Quite possibly her circumstances don't allow for what this might leave her with. Working on self harm brings up turmoil and unfinished business; a woman with a young family for instance is not in the best position to work on her vulnerabilities. Other life crises or pressures such as the lack of a secure home may also be relevant in determining her readiness to explore this area. Working towards damage limitation then is better during these times than giving up something which might be holding life together. If workers and counsellors were more open to allowing the woman to talk about self harm in a non judgemental way, it would help eliminate some of the guilt women carry about their actions. Sharing these things might even stop her harming on that occasion, or at least may prevent more severe injuries caused through added guilt and shame.

Workers and counsellors need to be clear on whether they feel able to cope with the painful feelings which may be aroused. Honesty on what can and cannot be tolerated is best discussed in early meetings if there is a possibility of self harm occurring. Having said that, injuries ARE frightening to observe; I often feel alarm and sometimes feel powerless to do anything other than offer first aid. HOWEVER, I wouldn't automatically assume control of the situation by getting the woman to show me her wounds. Women have had their bodies and lives invaded enough. I do not believe it is therapeutic to interfere further by trying to take away the only power she has at this present time. If she allows, I try to work with her in assessing whether she is in need of emergency treatment. Very often, the wounds are superficial, even though there is a lot of blood. Having someone who cares enough to want to share this painful reality can be therapeutic, a huge contrast to the anger and rejection she may well have encountered before.

I have heard from women who have begun their self harm during initial therapy sessions. Sometimes women have talked about a need to know the therapist's integrity and ability to give support in times of huge distress:

Anne: "I 've been going for psychotherapy for 80 weeks now. She is a good therapist but tough at times in the name of bitter REALITY. She gave me an overdose of facing bitter reality, the shadow self one session. I came home, scared and very ashamed of what she had uncovered, unable to cope until my next session the following week. I felt I was going mad. Cutting instantly eased my pain. I felt no shame for what I had done; I wasn't hurting anyone else or inconveniencing them, unlike an alcoholic friend of mine. As I smoothed Germolene on my cuts, I pretended that someone else was tenderly caring for me, not judging but saying "There, there, Anne" as one would to a child who had fallen over and hurt herself. My therapist does mother me WHEN SHE judges it appropriate. The lack of it in a longed for, precious and expensive once weekly session sends me frantic with anguish. I don't think she is the sole cause but she had triggered it off. I could compare it to a match being set to a slow burning fuse of unexpressed anger/longing over a very long time, or like a dentist's drill hitting an exposed nerve. When my therapist first saw my cuts she said it made her feel very sad, as she had tried to care for me. Perhaps by cutting myself I was trying to force her to admit some positive feelings towards me and not wear that so clinically, infuriatingly deadpan expression."

Marion: "I had three admissions to a psychiatric hospital for depression, and psychotherapy following my discharge. I understood about psychotherapy and that I would have to be very honest, think about my feelings towards others and my own feelings and resentments. BUT the intense, overwhelming anger, and the terrors that this brought to me, were definitely NOT expected. My psychologist stirred up a great deal of anger within me, and then left me to cope alone until my next appointment with her the following week. The anger built up and was really terrifying. There were no other outlets. I first made several superficial cuts to the top of my arm, and was quite surprised at what I had done."

There are dangers that therapy can trigger powerful feelings that may result in self harm. Exploring intense material can be extremely painful and frightening. At these times it is better if a woman can be supported in finding ways of nurturing herself and if possible enabled to take a step back from intensive work. Women have talked about drawing up strategies to plan out their days, perhaps carrying through simple tasks, or contacting people to "take off the pressure." Even staying in bed reading or sleeping can help. What is needed, even before things become too difficult (and therefore feel impossible to think about), are possible plans for getting through times such as these, and therapists can be of help in thinking about this.

The building of a trusting therapeutic relationship is essential, before any other work takes place. This process can take time to develop, especially as most women are used to being rejected for self harming . There may well be fears that the therapist will turn out to be yet another person who will 'intrude' and take control when she feels vulnerable and unprotected. Some therapies by their nature are intense and exploratory; a few women have found this work rather 'too invasive' of their space. It takes time for a woman to feel ready to discuss and work on her vulnerabilities; she needs to build up a level of trust first, or she simply may not find these kinds of approaches useful.

A counsellor's commitment to the woman's path of healing, her understanding and respect of those defence mechanisms - which take time to dismantle, need talking about in a way which values the part they have played in a woman's life. Therapies which work with a woman, at a pace she is comfortable with, such as humanistic or feminist approaches might be suggested - though unfortunately, due to the limitations of resources, most of these are found privately.

I want to include something about 'Cognitive Therapy' as a couple of women I talked to found this useful and were able to receive it through the NHS. This approach centres around exploring in detail thoughts and feelings which occur around difficulties, or as in this particular case, around the time of self harm. Theory tells us that people are then enabled to gain some recognition and understanding of what goes on at these times and learn to channel feelings in less harmful ways. Though it must be said women report finding this useful if they also have other support or therapy which recognises underlying processes and difficulties, on its own, it may not in any way be supportive enough of how women feel.

Helen writes: "I first used self harm as a method of expressing feelings seven years ago. I have no recollection of the first occasion or what triggered it. I do know that I used a hammer to beat the backs of my hands and the inside of my arms. The pain and bruising made it easier to bear the mental pain which was reaching horrendous proportions - at least the pain become visible. As time went on I found the sharp edges of the hammer could pierce the skin. The pain was sharper and more effective in establishing control over feelings inside. Over a year my depression deepened to a point where anguish was intolerable and I asked to be admitted to hospital. Whilst in hospital (despite much care which was good) there were instances when I felt intense frustration that my insights into my situation and needs were not considered relevant. It was after one conversation with a Senior Registrar that I picked up a plastic ash tray and slammed it against my arm. It cracked and as I repeatedly hit my arms with the piece in my hand, slashes appeared down my arms. The relief was enormous. The feeling was of unexpressed emotion streaming out of me for the first time in months - or years. It was a way at times of gaining control over my feelings and 'shocking me' out of depression so that I could get into work or undertake other activities. I stopped cutting for a couple of years but then my cutting escalated and I found it was necessary to cut ever more deeply to gain relief - with most relief obtained when I cut deep veins with a fast flow of blood. I also cut my legs and - to a limited extent - my neck."

Helen cont.: "I am fully aware of the dangers of this and regret the permanent damage I have caused to myself. The most helpful therapy I have received has been a cognitive approach (this was on the NHS). It was the only time anyone has ever asked me to describe in detail exactly what I did when cutting, what I was thinking and what I felt when cutting. (I have found that most psychiatrists or counsellors are interested in what triggers self harm, but not in the experience itself). I found it liberating that someone was prepared to enter with me into the experiences of cutting - to listen to the feelings and to ask for details which build a picture of the event. After conditioning myself to protect others from details which frighten or sicken them, it was an enormous surprise that someone wanted to know. Cognitive therapy itself involved looking in minute detail at the situations, thoughts and feelings which led up to cutting and exploring a range of responses and thoughts when I could 'choose' in a situation. At the time of therapy I was suffering from depression. This approach helped me - to a certain extent - manage the depression and - at times - avoid cutting.

However, I noticed greater benefit once the depression lifted. Then I could draw on the repertoire of techniques learnt in therapy to deal with situations which would have led to cutting in the past. The therapy has helped me gain a degree of choice - I know there is a variety of ways I can respond to a situation. Having said that, there were times when I believe that, for me, at the time, cutting was the only possible way of coming through an appalling emotional situation. Neither am I sure that cognitive therapy on its own would have helped me. I had already developed some understanding of why I self harm through exploration of adolescent relationships and psychotherapy (which was privately arranged). I am still re-learning how to express feelings - through painting, writing, my voice and movement - and that continues."

Behavioural changes in my opinion only have cosmetic value. If a woman has little or no self worth, she will be unable to gain much from this type of therapy. While it is encouraging when a woman says she has stopped harming, sooner or later she may return to this method of release, or, she might turn to other forms of self harm such as drugs or alcohol to numb or 'deaden' feelings of anger and hopelessness.

Learning to understand one's behaviour can be useful, but therapies which are solely behaviourally focused may lead women into the role of being the good client, doing what is expected, fearing a loss of support. Women are 'good' at looking after other people; many do not expect to be understood or have their needs met. Some have had their needs trampled on in childhood and have brutally learnt the necessity of following the wishes of an 'important other', probably having to 'lose' their feelings and themselves by 'forgetting' what life has really been like.

One could argue that techniques in modifying behaviour may only be useful in giving the therapist a sense of competence or control. We can feel good that we have achieved something and although it may be hard to admit, our own fears of helplessness are put back into manageable order.

I have spoken with workers, who, out of desperation or a belief that it will do some good, try to distract women through encouraging 'more positive behaviour.' Things such as needlework, sewing and other even household chores have been suggested to keep people 'occupied'. Personally, I think this attitude reflects the fears of those who are doing the suggesting; it certainly undermines and further disables women. There are no 'quick fix' methods of healing; being distracted from what is painful is what woman are used to. To be offered yet another distraction, further avoids the issue and says to her "I don't know how to deal with your pain. I am scared. Make me feel better." Women are resourceful; otherwise none would survive other people's dismissiveness and belittling of their pain!

Some may even question whether therapy is useful at all. What is the point of looking at what helps the individual, if that individual is merely reacting to oppressive life circumstances which do not change? That is something for each of us to answer for ourselves and decide what we need to do, if anything. The important point is that we understand how restrictive and abusive practices lead women to feeling powerless, and that self harm is the result of that powerlessness.

But we as counsellors can equally get caught up with feeling as powerless as the woman. It is worth giving thought to our own support when working with self harm. So let us look further at what we as workers may need for ourselves and then I'll discuss some of the questions workers have raised with me.

During training workshops with professional or voluntary groups, my colleagues and I have often asked people about what support they have and need. I find it startling how little support workers get, or expect to receive. Some may not even have a clear idea of what support means and talk about irregular supervision meetings where practical issues get discussed. Feelings, although often running high, are rarely disclosed in fear of reprisals. And there may be a sense of hopelessness about asking for anything more. But can we really care for someone else if we are not cared for ourselves? And if we cannot voice our feelings and needs, then how can we expect our clients to? There needs to be more support of a confidential kind within organisations. This might be mutual support, peer group or facilitated. It is SO important to have space and time to off-load on a regular basis. Perhaps then fewer staff would go off sick with stress related illnesses and would feel better and more effective in the good work they do. If organisations won't pay out, it is worth setting up one's own - our wellbeing deserves supporting surely? For anyone who works with self harm - good supervision/support is absolutely ESSENTIAL.

'Professionalism' does not make us immune to the stress we accumulate daily. It does not detach us from a world full of negative feelings and attitudes which pervade our lives both generally and in our work. This bombardment of unfulfilled needs and demands is draining of our energy. Add on top of this a situation where we find ourselves, at the end of a long hard day, supporting a woman who has come to us with self inflicted injuries - and our stress becomes intolerable. Feelings of anger rise as we experience the weight of our exhaustion and our inadequacy in that situation. How easy it then becomes to blame the woman for this added stress and even if we have no wish to be angry, we do feel angry! Honesty is best here; it is far better to admit you are unable to help at this moment in time and suggest a time when you might feel better able to support her, or suggest other agencies who might be more suitable if you cannot deal with her harming. It is important that workers look after their needs - otherwise they will hinder rather than help.

Perhaps on another occasion, we have been supporting a woman over a length of time and she turns up with wounds which are bleeding. Although we have been aware that she injures herself, she hasn't brought the subject up before and we haven't asked her about this. Do we say anything now and if we do, what might we say? If her injuries are that apparent, for instance on her hands, or we can see bloodstains, I would personally take this as a sign that she was wanting to talk about her self injury. As to what to say, well, what would you say to someone who had an accident and had come to you? You wouldn't ignore their injuries but would want to be gently talking with that person about how they felt and what had happened. Some believe that the need to harm will be reinforced through showing concern. But how many times do we as workers get sick in times of stress and want people to notice we are ill, show us kindness when we are feeling vulnerable? Few of us get the love and attention we deserve and we can easily slip into feeling this lack when faced with someone who is so obviously in need. There again, if we do raise the subject of self harm, we need to be ready to listen and carry on supporting her for as long as needed. Some workers may not want or be able to do this. Again it is O.K. to choose not to deal with self injury but instead support women in finding someone else who can work with them, although agencies may sometimes use self harm as a reason not to work with women. When resources are low, boundaries around who might be excluded become tighter. A woman who harms herself may be seen as too 'unstable' or "needy' if counselling can only be offered short term. While I think short term work may stir up more problems than can be resolved in the time given, can we really make gereralised judgments about women's needs? Do we exclude the women who admit to harming but see those who are less obvious in what they do? Each woman's needs and ability to cope with counselling would be better discussed with her and if it is the case that policies have to be made, it is worth explaining how this has come about.

Another question workers ask is what to do when a woman comes to us with what appears to be a heightening of her self injury. It goes through our minds that she might die and we could be held responsible. We want to do something, to act and save the situation. But are we really responsible for what someone else does to themselves? Do we have a legal or moral responsibility in preserving life or protecting someone against extreme damage? Workers from statutory organisations especially are faced with a dilemma on whether to take this further, working as they do within certain guidelines. In this case it is far better to be honest with the woman about these obligations, preferably having discussed these eventualities beforehand.

It may be useful to find out how long self harm has been going on. Is this something new? It may have been going on for years - yet she has survived thus far. Of course there is always a danger of fatality at some time now or in the future: tragic deaths do occur. But this possibility is just as true for any person in deep distress. They may die through their actions. One simply cannot predict what the outcome might be. If a woman has enough information about, for example, where her arteries are, or how different drugs can build up to toxic levels, she is better able to decide on the extent of damage she can inflict with the minimum of danger. What is probably as important is sharing with her this acutely painful time in her life that needs such drastic relief.

Stepping in and 'rescuing' someone from themselves is not a good course to be continually following. It disempowers rather than empowers a woman. We see someone in acute pain and want to make things better but the truth is we cannot make it better for anyone else. We can only share with her some of the weight of her experience and let her know our commitment to being with her through this. Her eventual healing will come through her finding her own strengths, and her own inner knowledge of what she needs, even if this is unclear right now.

We might ask ourselves what we expect of women who are engaged in harming. Are they really doing something so wrong? How would we cope given a similar set of circumstances? Would we do any better? Most of us strive to achieve some vague image of happiness and contentment which always seems beyond our grasp. Reality never quite meets the fantasy we so longingly seek. Maybe her method of coping is fine given the harsh reality. She is at least communicating something about how it feels.

Workers might worry that discussing feelings about death will heighten the probability of it happening - not so. These feelings need to be expressed and explored. Women often feel relief in being given the opportunity to talk without having the threat of someone panicking and perhaps enforcing sectioning or hospitalisation. Sometimes though, women who feel extremely powerless, especially those who already have experience of psychiatry may appear to place themselves where hospitalisation and or sectioning will result. Feeling painfully uncontained and unable to comprehend survival without it being enforced, they arrive again and again in the position of 'control' through force. Her needs during times of crisis for some holding containment would be better addressed outside of psychiatry or or institutions. But because as yet there is little in the way of crisis provision for women, a revolving door scheme in women only wards would at least allow women to come and go when they needed to. It would provide some safety - as long as women had absolute say over what happened to them. And so, when a psychiatric survivor seems to be asking for secure containment and feels this is her best choice right now, it is better to encourage her to be thinking about what she is needing from hospitalisation and explore ideas on how to go about getting some of those needs met. Making a voluntary admission is better than being sectioned.
Should we act as moral managers over women's decisions? For example, women who talk about wanting to end their lives are exercising their right to have control over their destiny. If we have given a woman space to talk over her feelings and needs and

she is fully informed of the choices available, in the end it is her life to decide over. While it's impossible to know whether a woman will go on to kill herself, perhaps having one person who is prepared to sit and listen will make a difference.

How empowering it is to have one's needs and feelings taken seriously without someone else panicking and taking control, to find someone who is prepared to listen and affirm the cruel ways life circumstances have robbed her of power and continue to make her feel vulnerable.

It may be good to explore the issue of power. The possibilities of how having power might effect changes in a woman's life can gradually enable her to begin challenging her position. We need to be aware also of the deep seated feelings and responses this can provoke: The child that was, the realisation that she was powerless in childhood and survived by having to endure whatever came her way. Self harm enable her to find some control over her suffering - but survival now has also become an endless endurance test of struggle and difficulty. These tests of strength may find voice through hours spent in self harming. Her wounds, the visible proof of her abilities, can give a measure of pride. And while her coping skills need recognition, at some point she may feel a need to begin the journey away from being on the 'cutting' edge of survival. And for this she needs to feel supported and affirmed as a woman who has found the strength and courage to survive thus far. She has the choices of an adult and will not be destroyed through experiencing her own power.

I have talked to workers who find women's increased anger hard to deal with. If woman express anger in an overt way, they may feel attacked by these seemingly 'inappropriate' outbursts which can appear to be directed at the worker. Here our old programming is telling us to defend ourselves from attack: our adrenalin drives us to want to take action. So we might get angry back. Then afterwards we feel guilty, our minds going over and over the situation, reprimanding ourselves for our own behaviour. Or we stay with the angry feelings and feel resentful or blaming. If, though, we were able to look beyond our own agendas at what is happening we might see something quite different. I am not suggesting that we overlook any abuse that is thrown at us. We do not have to take aggressive behaviour. But behind a woman's defences there is someone in acute pain - who is waiting for yet another person to hurt and reject her, who may through her fears set up a situation where this is exactly what does happen. I would personally point this out to a woman and try to work at identifying all the people in her life who have hurt and rejected her in the past. Her anger is very valid and necessary for healing. I show her that I am not rejecting her for being angry and if she is angry with me, I talk to her about that.

Counsellors often talk in depth about projections and transference issues, working on the assumption that any powerful feelings arising from the client are projections from her inner world. While I am clear that this, in part, is happening - maybe also there is something about my own responsibilities within a counselling relationship which needs addressing. It can be dismissive of personal responsibility to justify everything that goes on within a counselling relationship by talking only in terms of 'the client's transference'. We need to think about our own position as counsellors, the power imbalance, which to some extent or another will be an issue within a counselling setting. Also, I think it is worth talking to women about anger, giving validity to the difficulties women encounter generally.

I have worked in women's hostels and have worked with staff from residential units where often self harm is an unspoken issue which generates anger amongst residents and concern amongst staff. One woman is seen to be receiving all the attention, which can create demands or crises between women. This is a particularly difficult situation to handle when staffing levels are low and perhaps it is down to one worker on shift to understand and work with the different dynamics going on. Each woman has a need for the small amount of attention there is to go around but has difficulty in verbalising these needs. Women may well feel guilty for their neediness and fearful that they may have their requests in asking for time rejected. This generates tension and unvoiced anger. Any woman at this point who finds a way to express her needs becomes the target for everyone's feelings. For example, the self harming woman becomes a focus for anger and blame, Staff may then attempt to restore order through also blaming and dismissing her actions as 'attention seeking,' or may 'rescue' her to the exclusion of others. I'm afraid there are no easy solutions here but being realistic about the impossibility of really meeting anyone's needs in difficult situations might be discussed and shared with colleagues and funding agencies. There needs to be enough staff, especially during evenings and weekends when crises tend to occur rapidly. Also I have found it useful to discuss self harm with the women and how we all express our needs for attention in different ways, and the difficulties of asking for time when others seem to be more needy and ways of going about getting some of these needs met. I think it is good to suggest other agencies or groups who can offer support and have this kind of information readily available. There is only so much we can do when we are short of valuable resources and we are human being who have our own limitations.

Sometimes the question of women using multiple agencies come up during training sessions. Is it O.K. to be using more than one agency or service, or would it be better if the work were consolidated and the woman were supported by one person alone? I think the woman has enough knowledge of her needs to know what is best for her at any given time, It may be too difficult to trust one person with all her painful material. And at first taking small risks with a few different people can be a testing out of who works well with her and can be trusted with information . I believe counsellors can become too 'precious' with their clients - don't most of us have different friends with whom we share varying levels of different information about ourselves? Of course there is a danger that too much spreading of material can overly fragment the healing process in the longer term. But certainly in the beginning at least I think having different people is useful. Especially as most workers are limited in time and women's needs may be huge, I think it can be useful all round to know women have other supporters.

Another point which I think is important is the danger of assuming an absence of self injury is a sign of improvement and responding to this by withdrawing the level of support. Whilst it is good that the woman has been able to go for a length of time without harming, it is very unwise to level off the support at this time of acute vulnerability. If anything, women need more support at this time as they deal with the acutely painful material which surfaces as a result.

There are no right answers, no right ways of working; what is important though is the therapeutic relationship itself and a commitment on both sides to working through difficulties. One important piece of information I'd like to share if you fall into the trap of feeling inadequate or hopeless in what you do: A friend of mine once told me that throughout her abusive childhood she had no supportive carers, no one to listen to her and was shunted around various institutions. One thing stuck in her memory, though, on one occasion she was sent to a foster home for one week. Although as she said 'nothing special happened' her foster mother during that short time listened to her without judgement and showed warm concern for her welfare. She said she had never forgotten this and although it didn't change her life much at that time, it provided her with the knowledge of being worth something and this gave her strength to cope with many other difficulties. Eventually she went on to seek therapy and is now a strong and powerful woman. Even when we can't see any, if all we do is listen and show that we care - there is hope!

ANGRY WOMAN

Angry woman rising
Flying above the struggle and pain.
- No more awash in a sea of bloody tears
    Will I waste my time.

    See me rising

        I am shouting

            I am singing

    I am dancing to my own song

        Mary (1994)

I would now like to share with you some of my own story and then go on to include something from Pat, (my friend and colleague) and will bring in some of my other contributors' stories.

SECTION SIX

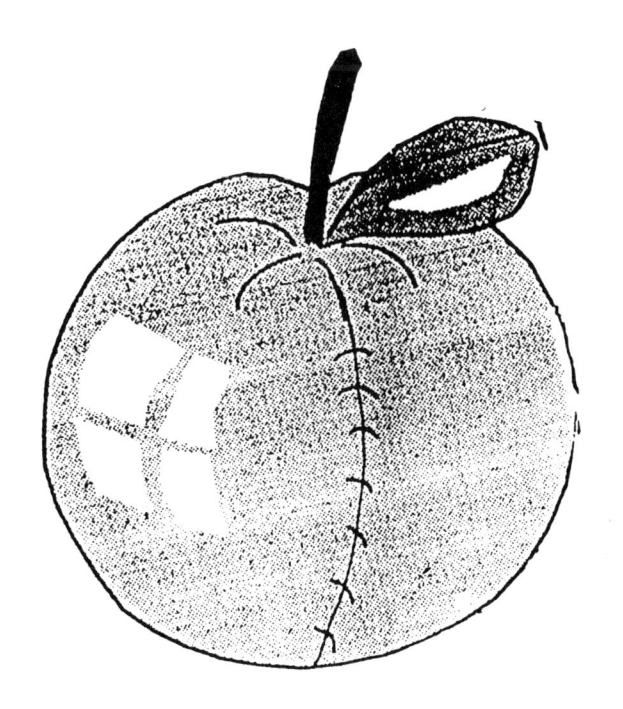

PERSONAL EXPERIENCES - Journeys of survival

DIANE HARRISON

THE JOURNEY

My own self harm began when I was very young and continued well into my thirties. I can safely say this kept me alive, sane, in a world full of unspoken confusion and mistruths.

I had been abused since early childhood by my grandfather, He was a vicar, who every Sunday would preach morality from his pulpit. For the rest of the week he might have acted out his own version of hell, but on Sundays he became self righteous and 'Godly.'

Self harm was my coping mechanism, it helped me survive childhood. The only way I could cope with being in my body was by emotionally and mentally dissociating myself from it. I felt as if my body had betrayed me by attracting so much 'evilness' into it and that if I had been a better child it would not have happened.

I lived with my parents and grandparents in the vicarage until I was 5 years old. It was a big rambling place, dark, with many rooms. I would run around trying to find each member of my family as they distanced themselves from each other in various corners of the house, meeting only at mealtimes. The vicarage grounds, though, gave me much pleasure and I would spend hours playing outside - largely on my own except when my grandmother came out to sing to me and push me on my swing. But indoors it was different; I remember a lot of arguments and conflict between people and feeling like I had to somehow keep the family together. I felt invisible, overlooked amongst everyone else's needs.

I began hurting myself because it made sense of the confusion and pain I experienced but was unable to voice. Sometimes I would hurt myself to prove that it existed. The sight of blood was exciting; it was something I could control. Cutting or scratching myself with twigs or whatever I could find mattered a lot to me. I could care for my wounds, look after them and make them better. This eased for a while my emotional pain.

If anyone asked about my injuries, I was expert in telling stories about my 'accidents' in detail. In that way I could get other people to give me the attention I needed. My physical wounds would then be looked after, even if my emotional pain remained raw and neglected. I hated my body; it seemed to have betrayed me by looking so innocent. I wanted to tear it to shreds, so that it spoke of the real truth and was punished.

By now we had moved away from the vicarage but I still saw my grandfather regularly. I loved him because he gave me attention. No matter what that attention had come to entail, it was important and reached me on some level. I felt emotionally cut off from the outside world; my inner world was in turmoil. I desperately wanted to feel loved and warm yet I felt cold and terribly alone. How sad, I had no one to listen to my conflicting feelings, make them real by validating their existence. I had no one to confirm the reality of abuse. So I hurt myself to save me from the insanity of the sheer pretence of it all. Life seemed to be about dressing up and telling the world that all was well, like wearing a mask that doesn't really fit and feels uncomfortable but having to wear it anyway. What was underneath, the reality, was denied in favour of the surface camouflage.

I felt treated differently from the rest of my family. I was 'special' to my grandfather, yet seemed to carry the pain of everyone's feeling on my small shoulders. The scapegoat for unspoken family guilt, I was denied my real needs and after my two sisters were born, this difference grew. I heard I was the odd one out, never quite matching up to anyone else. I duly responded to these messages by failing miserably at school, never quite coming up to grade; except, though, in art, my creativity was always prolific; I seemed to be able to express life through my paintings. I saw the vivid colours of nature in my mind's eye, the reflections of a life that I had experienced in earlier childhood. Just as I had once loved running free through the fields surrounding vicarage grounds, so I now loved the freedom of expression art provided me, though, If I produced a particularly good picture because I felt so undeserving of anything nice, I often hurt myself to bring me back from my euphoric state.

Survival seemed to depend on experiencing little in the way of emotions or feelings. Even the messages I got about being female told me to be 'ladylike', quietly smiling, suffering in silence if necessary, always giving with no expectations of receiving back. Achieving beauty meant acceptance into the world and for this sacrifices had to be made. As a teenager I watched my friends go on diets in the name of fashion. This was in the sixties when everyone wanted to look like Twiggy and wear mini skirts. To be accepted into 'the gang' at my school you had to appear to be following the fashion trends laid down in the popular magazines. One friend went on a diet and became anorexic; others trussed themselves up in corsets to diminish in size and had to suffer hours of discomfort and pain. But these forms of self harm were upheld as 'normal' behaviours, especially for young girls. The belief in reducing one's size and shape, altering one's looks was freely discussed in the playground and was reinforced by the messages in the adult media. I went along with this just to feel accepted by my peers, but sometimes during increasing periods of depression I cut myself 'secretly' to express my inner fury at the world. I didn't fit; I didn't particularly want to fit into this preconditioned mould.

Grandfather died when I was 16. I felt guilty for his death and missed him dreadfully. I took an overdose, not because I wanted to die; I just wanted life to change. It did; it gave me the spark to leave home and go abroad for a while. It also had the effect of erasing past memories. I simply forgot my childhood and if something reminded me, I cut myself severely to try and forget it again.

At 18 I started training to become a nurse. I loved nursing but hated looking after the older men; they reminded me of something but I could not remember what. Although I was able to hold myself together on the ward, after work I would race back to my small room in the nurses' home and cut my body to erase overwhelming visions that seemed to leap out at me. I hated my body; I hated inhabiting it. I was not suicidal, though; it was as if dying was beyond me. To have wanted to die I should have had to have felt something and I was far away from feeling anything that strongly.

A few times I ended up in casualty, where I told stories about my 'accidents', which seemed to satisfy staff. I would not have dared to have said anything different and looking back, I am glad I did not. Nobody knew anything about self harm back in the 70's and even now in the 90's little is understood. Not only would I have been labelled 'mad' or 'bad', I could have been struck off the register - and little has changed to this day I am afraid. As I sit and write now I have a whole pile of letters beside me from nursing staff who are in fear of their jobs, or who have already been struck off for a wide range of harming 'behaviour' from eating distress to self injury.

There was this need in me to care for others - as much as I wanted to be cared for, I see now - and I gave great attention to my patients' needs. As a female I had been well groomed into the role of carer and I really enjoyed my work. Being an abuse survivor I was finely 'tuned' into noticing situations, able to notice problems even before they occurred. This intuitive 'knowing' gave me a good reputation amongst colleagues, where I was classed as a highly competent nurse.

I was even a highly competent housewife and mother when I got married, though I have to admit with my first daughter I found my feelings in turmoil. She reminded me of myself as a child and this was too much to bear. I wanted to hurt her but felt guilt for having these feelings and hurt myself as punishment. Gradually I found my emotionally immature husband too difficult, too. His needs for attention and his demands for sex began to remind me of the past. To deal with this I took up a writing course and wrote essays at bedtime, creeping into bed in the early hours of the morning, long after my husband was asleep. It is strange to remember the stories I wrote. They held an element of the truth in them although I believed they were fictional. All of them said something about my past - like an emotional one I wrote about a dying child. Several others were mystery suspense or ghost stories. Possibly each could have identified my haunted past, parts of my life which were yet to surface and become real for me.

My husband left me eventually. We had by now been married 7 years and had produced 3 children, all under 5 years old. I felt abandoned and guilty for having failed. Depression crept in and I was unable to cope so was given antidepressants by my doctor and a social worker.

I became very bulimic and thin. In throwing up I was chucking up my disgust at the world. At least at this time I was just beginning to say 'no' to the things I no longer could digest. In the past I just said 'yes' and digested anything that was given to me. So in this sense there was a marked change, though my doctor thought I was getting much worse and referred me to a psychiatrist.

I wanted to talk and have some support yet I saw the psychiatrist only once. He told me that I was lucky to be receiving help at all (think it was pull yourself together time). I became very upset and was admitted to hospital a few weeks later with the label 'reactive depression.' More pills and some O.T. were tried with little success. So the labels mounted up like badges: 'hysterical', 'attention seeking', 'neurotic', 'histrionic' and that I was 'trying to manipulatively get my husband back.' Actually, I was very distressed, in need of attention, would try hard to get something - except not from my husband; I did not want him back!

I was self harming a lot in those days and on one visit my social worker confronted me about this. She seemed concerned about the effect it might have on the children if they found out. I admitted harming but told her of the trouble I went to in protecting my children from what I had done. Then all of a sudden it poured out of my mouth, "I was abused as a child." She gave me 6 weeks of counselling and then left me to get on with it - but I felt like I had taken the lid off from something massive which could destroy me. My self harm increased and I had several further admissions to hospital, where eventually I lost custody of my children to their father.

I was devastated; my world had fallen apart. I was kept on the locked ward to keep me safe. Yet it was not safe; it was full of men, one of whom made several advances at me. On one occasion when he approached me talking about sex, I burnt my hands with a cigarette, I was so scared. At least this way I could distance myself from my feelings enough not to care what happened. I am not sure now what did happen. I can only remember the staff getting angry and disbelieving me about the seriousness of what had gone on.

One male psychiatric nurse took me on board as 'his' case and spent his time ridiculing me. One day he told me I'd look better if I plucked my eyebrows and put on make-up, so in my defiance I picked up a piece of glass and cut patterns into my face. It was my only way of saying 'fuck off' to my keepers - but my punishment was in being ignored until I cooled down and would talk to staff about how I felt. I couldn't; I didn't have the words to explain; I didn't trust these people anyway. There was no reason to trust them with such powerful feelings when they wouldn't try to understand my language of communication, believe how unsafe I felt.

Eventually I pretended to play their game by muttering a few lines every day and they let me out. It took me a few more visits before I realised that for me, hospitalisation was a damaging way of revictimizing myself to powerful others. I had wanted a place of safety, not to feel threatened and to fear further abuse in whatever way it arrived.

I took control by moving into a supportive women's hostel where I received twice weekly counselling. This was much better; I was at least being believed and taken seriously. Yet before looking at my childhood and beginning to explore my feelings, I had to work through the damage caused through the 'treatment' I had received thus far. It took a very long time to learn to trust someone enough with my feelings to let them in. It took even longer for me to learn that my feelings wouldn't destroy me or cause something 'bad' to happen. My hope is that the women who were involved in these years of my neediness will learn how valuable they were to me and my healing. At times I know I tested them and gave them a very hard time but they were valuable witnesses to the toughness of my journey and I will never forget them.

Self harm continued for me until I was ready to let go of it. When I had more understanding of what was inside and was real (my inner world) there was no need to go digging to prove I existed. My experiences happened and through becoming involved in feminism and counselling I had understood them in context. They were not extraordinary to me and neither was the way I reacted to them. My body now is covered in scars but in a way I feel proud of them. Each one seems to mark out a battle I had with life and got through, survived. What strangely 'creative' things we find to survive and express our desperation. How sad that we have to do so.

For the last few year I have been involved in training professional and voluntary groups and have worked in women's support groups. At the moment, apart from training work, I am working with a few women on an individual basis.

I have learnt so much from my journey and have witnessed so much pain, being and now working quite literally at times at the knife edge of survival. But I feel hugely hopeful and excited at just being alive and at seeing others make the leap into life and freedom. As my colleague Pat said to me recently "The best way I have found of getting back at my abuser is now having a good life and enjoying myself." I agree, I have stopped doing a sentence for the crimes that were imposed on me as a child and I am free to live and have choices.

I would like to end this piece by including something rather precious to me. Creativity has featured much in my healing and I have painted pictures, written and even danced and sung my way through the rough road of healing. This particular letter I wrote as I took the first steps towards learning to love my inner child self. You might say that I wrote it as I gave birth to her. It was a difficult delivery and at first I wasn't sure that I could cope with this new child! But I kept her anyway and she has grown into something very beautiful and strong.

My Dearest Child   (written in 1992)

This is the first time I've been able to address you and call your name. Never before have I been able to think of you in these terms 'my' 'dearest'. I used to hate you, despise the fact that you were me, inside me. I wanted to abandon your presence or push you onto someone else who could heal you, look after your needs or simply abuse you some more. I didn't care, I just wanted you out of my life.

Now I can look back and remember the person you were, before your childhood was ripped away -the little girl who loved to sing and dance in the meadows with the sun and wind in her hair, dancing and embracing nature and life itself. You were free then; every moment brought forth the excitement of learning and experiencing new joys and pleasures, like the time when you climbed up onto the table at Christmas and sang 'The Lord's My Shepherd'. Your audience clapped with pleasure watching you draped in a sheet, clutching closely a lighted candle, trying to mimic the choir at church. The adults couldn't fail to notice the light and life in those big blue eyes, the pure energy of blossoming youth.

No one noticed you slip away only weeks later, to be replaced by a quiet lost child with haunted eyes. The trust that you'd given so freely was withdrawn to all when your most trusted friend, grandfather, abused your tiny body and wounded your mind and spirit when he taught you
 secrets and unholy death if you disobeyed.

He had been your hero, the God-like vicar who preached damnation to all sinners, who had fed you with goodness and the warmth of pure heaven. Now you felt like a sinner, doing penance for a crime you couldn't understand. You believed that you had drawn too much attention to being yourself. Bad and tainted flesh, you had inherited the devil into your blood and veins.

In terror you fled from your body by night in case it was further hurt, or let itself down by screaming out the nightmares of waking sleep. No one could hear you; your family were locked into their own prisons of struggle. The only way of releasing those screams were by scratching or even cutting them out, watching the blood pour away the evil you felt inside.

Dearest child, it has taken me years to hold you, reach you and mother your rights to be free and yourself, to reclaim you from that lonely land of dreams where only unholy death or madness lay. I had to reach out my hand across the pain of many years to where you existed in your misty grey hell, and sit with you, walk with you, be with you in that lonely place, keep you close to me even though I couldn't always listen to your screams, nor feel your intense pain.

It's still holding your hand. It's no longer a trial to do so; it's a pleasure. I feel too proud of that fragmented spirit who has determined not to lie down and let death nor never ending madness overcome life. That little soldier spirit won her battle. She is the precious, joyful and creative part of myself - My dearest child.

Pat Hagen

"I see my self harm as a long journey. When I was little I created accidents, like trying to jump out in from of a milk float - but I was little and couldn't judge the distance and it stopped halfway down the road! I used to fall off my bike, and once cut my fingers by accident. When cutting an orange I nearly cut the top off and I've still got that scar. I was fascinated by blood. I was about 11 then but I was always falling over. But actually I didn't need to do much to myself, because my mum was pretty violent and so was my dad.

I was proud of my bruises. I think if I'd actually done them myself it might have been different but it was very much an outward sign of what was going on inside, total confusion. I couldn't understand why people accepted it and did nothing about it, or ask why I was bruised. I was happier at school; it was my escape because I didn't know how to talk to people, how to make friends. At home no one wanted to talk and wanted to push everything aside - the favourite one was 'What would the neighbours say, you can"t tell anyone anything'. I got pregnant at 14 and had to wear corsets when I came home from approved school so no one would see the bump. There was nothing real; the reality I was experiencing was completely mismatched with what was really going on. It's terrifying still to think of it. Self harm was a way of controlling it and a way of making myself feel something real. Once I'd had an accident or had hurt myself I'd be pulling the scabs off and I can see now that it was a way of looking inside to pull the covers off. It was certainly a world out of control for me, a frightening world but I only actively began self harming, I mean by that an active campaign, when I was 17. My father used to drink a lot and I had been drinking since I was 6. Alcohol was freely available in the house, I think I drank to be numb. It was a way of getting through the day; I had a huge feeling that I was different to everyone else. I could hardly speak, just the odd word but lived in my head with school work until I was 13. Then I tried to tell someone at school was was going on; they didn't believe me.

Up until I was 12 the self harm as 'accidental', then I started drinking heavily and got into abusive relationships, quite deliberately and in a way, numbing out as well. I was trying to cover everything up. I listened to the lies being said about me, that I was bad and dangerous and it was my fault. That started with my dad and mum and the social services, doctors and psychiatrist, anyone who had any power over me. Basically I was labelled a psychopath because I showed no deep emotions or guilt for what I had done to my patents. No one asked why I couldn't feel anything and I believed all this for years and tried hard to feel something, but couldn't.

At 17 I got out of care and had another baby but after 6 months I blew it and I was in the loony bin by the time the baby was 4 months old. I was drinking again and was drunk all the time. I was labelled as post-natally depressed; it was self neglect, but I kept myself just alive because I didn't want to die. The doctor gave me some pills and it was only when I took an overdose of them that he told me they were vitamin C and laughed at me. He didn't take me seriously and there was nowhere to go for help. I wanted someone to listen to me. I ended up back in the loony bin and what helped was the informal patient network. I made a friend of one woman and we had a lot of fun. I laughed for the first time in my life. We lived dangerously on the edge, I learnt to control my self harm to just the right degree. I could take just enough tablets to knock myself out but not enough to die. I just slid through this time in a haze and ignored the doctors who threw me out eventually, But I had to go and face reality again by which point my husband had left me and my children were in care.

But the self harm became more dangerous. Life was really on the edge. I'd take overdoses and was only by chance found. Also I was obsessively cleaning myself, bathed two or three times a day using bleach to clean myself. I used after shave and perfume on my genitals which burnt me but made me feel cleaner on the inside. I knew these things were crazy, I kept them secret but feared being smelly and going to the doctors.

These horrible cleansing rituals were to cleanse myself because I felt so dirty. I think I was at this point quite suicidal. I felt I was so dirty, abnormal, felt my life was over. I don't know how I stopped and moved on. I stopped drinking and began abusing prescribed drugs and having abusive relationships. I had my son back and that helped but I went into this dead phase and when the numbness wore off, I self harmed. It always went in waves. I wanted to be so-called normal, which stopped me drinking.

It's not just having the kids with me that helped. I don't know what it was but I moved in with a man who did all sorts of things. Because I was so out of touch with my body I didn't know when to eat or sleep. He was controlling but I felt he cared about me. As long as I was unable to make decisions he was O.K. but as soon as I tried to take control of my life he didn't like it, so I numbed off again. I was suicidal. I didn't feel there was anything else for me but when I self harmed, at least I did it for myself. It was more satisfying. I used to provoke danger; it was powerful. He hit me. I wanted him to because I'd feel something. I liked driving with people who drove fast. I even got into politics and went on demos and got beaten up several times. I wasn't into anything passive, I was living on the edge on picket lines! It was socially sanctioned within the group that I was in, encouraged; I really got a buzz from it. It was a most basic resistance. It's my body and I can do what I want with it. Not eating too was a good one. Not being able to get out of the chair even, because I was starving but just doing it anyway was saying 'it's my body and just keeping it alive, just for a bit longer.' But it went out of control and I provoked this bloke once too often and he nearly killed me. I was very lucky I got out of it and this moved me on to doing something.

I moved into meeting with other women and just talking about real things that made sense helped. My active self harming stopped apart from one last ditch attempt at an overdose. I still was far away from feeling good about myself and understanding what was going on but I never tried to risk my life again, though I did get into other abusive relationships and went into the caring professions where I got some buzz from helping others. That was a good substitute for a while and is socially sanctioned! I got into helping other people through advice work - constant trauma, I got very involved. Another form of self harm for me was pushing myself too much, not giving myself a break and felt I had to do things. I was a nervous wreck.

I don't have these adrenalin rushes now. I'm older and want to feel settled. I don't need to put myself into danger anymore. I realise that the more I got myself into danger and messed up my life the more my father won. My self harm was a necessary resistance to the abuse but now I have a better one - I can enjoy life and have fun. If I self harm these days it's in enjoyable ways. I choose to drink sometimes but it's much more of a life than I hoped for. I look back now and I can see that the breakthrough for me was when I realised my self harm was a coping mechanism, rather than was self destructive. It was a huge turning point. I realised that I did really want to live. It was a horrible realisation and I remember pacing the floor not knowing what to do but staying with my feeling and not doing anything about it. I stayed up all night. It was terrifying but I desperately wanted to get through it. Mostly the feelings were of anger and hate. It used to be me who I hated, now I was angry at the people who had done things to me. Things changed when I met other people who'd experienced this but generally I was beginning to question things in my life. I found a homeopath who listened and prescribed remedies which helped. It was a combination of many things for me at that time. The distance between what had happened to me was far enough away. I felt safer away from my family reminders My family always acted as if nothing had happened; it was so confusing. No one was saying anything beyond surface family issues. I thought that if I believed their version of what happened to me as a child they would hate me and not want to talk to me and if I believed my version, I should hate them and not want to talk to them. So I ended contact and that helped. I just couldn't relate in any real way to them with love or with hate. It didn't make sense. Since then I have spent lots of time working things out for myself.

REALITY TRIP

The trees are
Gently weeping in
Sympathy

As little droplets
Flow like blood
From a vein

Climax

Seeking permission
To vacate

No tears
Hard knot inside

The knife cuts
And the blood pours

No mercy, no surrender

Welcome.

Alex B   (1993)

LAUREN

My personal experience of self harm dates back about 4 years: 9 years if you count various bouts of eating disorders. I began cutting myself at the age of 21, starting with a kitchen knife and later graduating to razors and broken glass, I see the cause of my cutting as twofold, stemming from my inability to express feelings, particularly those of a 'dangerous' nature (i.e. anger, especially towards people close to me) due to early experience within my family of punitive response to the expression of anger or discontent, coupled with the sexual, physical and psychological abuse to which I was subjected by my stepfather.

Cutting serves two purposes for me; it relieves my feelings of anger and despair and also expresses in the form of injuries, the emotions I feel unable or too disempowered to express. I am aware that it is linked to my feelings of self-hate and disgust stemming from my abuse, and I believe these factors have contributed to my continuing choices of supportive and sensitive (or NOT) partners. Their reactions to my self harming have been varied; to be fair (not a habit of mine where men are concerned), some have attempted some degree of sensitivity and understanding, but most have taken a heavy handed, controlling approach, such as the immortal words of one of my ex-partners: "If you do that again, I'm going to have you fucking sectioned." Others have taken a judgemental and dismissive approach, "Do you do it to get attention? Of course I do. That's why I wear a sweat-shirt in the middle of August. No, no, you dance on a table in a crowded pub "to get attention." You do not hack up your body with a razor for the sole purpose of attracting attention.

This brings me to the subject of one of the most popular myths concerning self harmers, namely that we're all a bunch of attention seekers who need to grow up. It is this labelling process which is largely responsible for the dismissive attitudes that self harmers are often faced with; however, I personally feel that the cause is rooted a lot deeper than this.

The logical progression of this theory of 'attention seeking' would be for society to consider what it is that we are actually trying to draw attention to. Funnily enough, this rarely happens and thus self harmers tend to be trivialised and consequently disregarded. The knock on effect of this conspiracy of silence is that self harmers are pathologised and as a result feel obliged to hide their injuries. Why is this? Are we really a more offensive sight than say, a burns victim? Indeed, I have often wondered whether friends have helped me to cover up in order to spare my discomfort - or their own?

As a survivor, my scars are my way of expressing the emotional pain and anger I feel as a result of my abuse, feelings that I often feel unable to vocalise having been shamed and intimidated into silence by my abuser. Increasingly, the medical and psychological professions are becoming aware that acts of self harm are very often rooted in sexual abuse, and this fact is starting to be reluctantly acknowledged by the media and society. However, as many of us are aware, adult survivors of sexual abuse are not a very trendy cause to support, and therefore I would guess that the cover-up job surrounding the issue of self harm serves two main purposes. Firstly, it denies survivors a route (sometimes their only route) of self expression. Secondly, most of society quite simply can't cope with the issue of sexual abuse. (Case in point: Mr. "Do you do it for attention?", in receiving an awkward question, namely why do I cut myself, responded with "You're getting too heavy man! Chill out!" He then went on to suggest that next time I felt under stress, I should confide in him rather than cutting myself!?). Way to go. Dismiss the subject out of hand and you don't have to deal with it at all. Leave it to the survivors to sort it out by themselves; after all, they've had years of practice.

AND YOU WONDER WHY WE CUT OURSELVES!

IGNORANCE

I don't want to be any trouble
Don't worry about me, I'll be fine
I'd really like to talk to you
But I realise this isn't the time.

I won't make you listen to my whining
Wouldn't want you to think I'm a bore
I promise not to bleed on your duvet
Or vomit up pills on your floor.

Well, thanks for the loan of your jumper
For sparing me any shame
Thanks for treating me like an embarrassment
Thanks for ignoring my pain.

Ignorant people, so quick to judge
Knowing nothing about self harm
You say I do it for attention
So why do I cover my arms?

All you know is your own assumptions
What would you know of abuse?
You're quick to write me off as neurotic
Well, how about facing the truth?

My scars speak of the inner damage
Society tells me to hide
The scars on my body are ugly and painful
They mirror the scarring inside.

Lauren

ANON

When I started harming myself, I wasn't really aware of the reasons why, and I certainly didn't think about the fact that it might have been 'wrong' or strange 'behaviour'. I did get asked why I kept having 'accidents' but the truthful answer was that I didn't know. I was only about 14.

By the time I'd left home and gone to college, I realised that what I'd been doing was a bit scarey, but continued to play with matches. The burns were comforting. When I did them they didn't hurt, but I appreciated the familiar aching that followed as they healed up. It was a focus for my thoughts, distracting from other things that were going on. As college got even more stressful, the self harming got worse but I never actually thought about a correlation between these events; only when a counsellor suggested I do something very definite to help (take a year out) did I realise that things were going wrong. I was scared, and stopped self harming, visibly at least. I cannot remember how I coped but a combination of alcohol, sex and overwork got my degree. I am immensely grateful that I stuck at the course, but in truth I was too frightened to do anything else that might have dealt with whatever was going wrong. I didn't have the courage to do anything unorthodox, which would have caused great problems with my parents and made my life more difficult. It's no coincidence now, six years later, when I no longer have my parents, that I'm more able to deal with the self harm. I'm much more scarred but less scared. I also have a career (even if it feels like a farce because some days I feel far too inadequate to cope) and support networks (professionals and friends who don't wobble or run if you ask them to listen). I feel like I have a basis from which to work, to be alive, and most importantly, to feel. I know I have been very much influenced by my upbringing that I should fit into middle class more, and outwardly I have done that; inwardly now I have the security to face the mess I am.

And I would actually argue that I'm no worse a mess than most people. I am glad that my own coping mechanism has left me with visible reminders of the struggle and pain. I haven't destroyed my inner body with drugs. I can see exactly what I've done. And that says a lot about my need to control. With cutting and burning I have been able to contact feelings in myself when things have been going crazy. If I cannot cope, self harm helps me; my attention is focussed onto something I am familiar with (my body). The blood or the blisters hypnotically take me out of whatever it is I cannot face externally. The process of cleaning up and caring for the wounds is very much part of it; and if I'm lucky and they need attention (from myself) for a few days, then I am less likely to self harm again.

There is one major problem though; having taken years to acknowledge this cycle of "block off - cut/burn - feel better" it now doesn't work so well - I've seen through what I'm doing. I still want, need, to self harm; it just doesn't work so well for me and I have to accept that I need to see through the start of it all: the blocking off itself.

I CRY RED

Can I trust you with a secret?
Dare I break my isolation?
I hope you'll try to understand me
I cannot risk your condemnation.

I must be careful who I trust
Too many times I've been betrayed
There's very few things I have faith in
But I can trust my blade.

Blade's my comfort and support
The only thing I can rely on
Never too busy, she's always there
When I need a shoulder to cry on.

Imprisoned in my little shell
I cry my private tears
They flow from my body, not my eyes
I cry red, not clear.

Split my skin, release my blood
Free my despair and violence
The only way that I know how
I dare not break my silence.

What was done to me was wrong
But there's nothing wrong with me
The real damage damage lies within
In wounds that you can't see.

Lauren

LINDA

Many adults can look back on their childhoods with happy memories of fun, laughter and love. I cannot do that due to the physical and sexual abuse by my father, my father's friend and his wife.

It started at the age of three and ended in 1979 when my father died. Being forced to have sexual intercourse at this age was very painful both physically and emotionally. To lie in bed and hear him coming was hell. His sweating body and lingering cigarette smoke filling the room and my nose. I just wanted to be sick and for the bed to swallow me up. And all the time he said that he loved me and what he was doing to me was okay - after all he was my father.

He started to take me to see one of his friends. At first I enjoyed going there until one day his wife sat beside me and put her arms around my shoulders and her hands between my legs. I looked at my father for help; he just looked at me and smiled and told his friend's wife to carry on. It was okay. I wanted to die in disbelief; I couldn't believe what I was hearing. I was taken round there once a month only to be forced into oral and anal sex.

For three years I accepted what was happening to me. I couldn't go to anyone to tell because of the threats from my father. One of his punishments was to fill the bath with ice water and force me naked into the bath and hold me in until I agreed to let him do whatever he liked to me.

At the age of six the emotional pain became so great that all I wanted to do was to end all the pain. I hit the wall in my bedroom and all the emotional pain just went. For the first time I had found relief from this kind of pain. I found the physical pain of self harming became a normal part of my life. I found myself at school deliberately hurting myself, falling over in the playground or falling off apparatus in the gym. Doing this, I found, relieved the emotional pain and I received the warmth, love and attention that I had been looking for.

At the age of fifteen my father made me pregnant. I was told that I was going to have twins. Amy died a few hours after she was born due to the deformity she suffered. Gary was a goodlooking and healthy boy. I stayed with friends after he was born and when he was four months old my father just turned up and took him. I was out at the time. I felt so much anger, pain and guilt. The one thing that had belonged to me had been taken. The emotional pain was so over powering, I just couldn't stop myself from self harming. I took tablets, alcohol and cut both my wrists. I was found and taken to hospital. I was put into a psychiatric unit where I found the doctors were unsympathetic and not very understanding about why I was self harming. They told me that I was wasting their time and taking up a bed that someone else could be using. They did nothing to try to stop my self harming in any way whatsoever.

The hospital sent me to one of their hostels. I befriended someone called Chris. We used to go for drinks. Nothing else ever happened. Then one evening we met up with three of his friends. At the end of the evening I was forced into the back of Chris's van and I was repeatedly raped. The physical and emotional pain was so great I wished at the time that they would kill me to save me from all the pain I had to endure. Once back at the hostel, Chris said that he would kill me if I told anyone what he and his friends had done. The pain inside me just seemed to grow and grow. I had to stop it in some way. Then I started to realise that every time I self harmed I was trying to cut out all the bad inside me, most of all my father.

I am forty-one years old and I married for the first time in 1982. The marriage broke down after two years. The emotional pain of not being able to stay married, followed by guilt, anger and failure in everything I seem to have done, led me to turn to drink once again. I also cut my wrists again. Then I found that the emotional and physical pain I was feeling became directed at my husband . . . and I tried to kill him with a knife. I was so drunk at the time that I didn't even scratch him. Instead he pushed me down the stairs and I ended up in hospital for several days - I was very lucky to have survived.

I remarried in 1989. I have two children, a girl of four and a son aged two. For the first two years the marriage was great but things started to go wrong after the birth of my son. I tried to smother him when he was three months old. I was told that I was suffering from post natal depression. However, after a few months I started to realise that it wasn't that after all. It was the emotional pain left by my father and other past experiences. For over twenty years all of my past memories had been pushed to the back of my mind; the birth of my son triggered off some of the inward emotions. I knew then that I had survived the physical pain and that time had come to survive the emotional pain. I am still self harming, trying to come to terms with the past. I have recently found out that my mother knew of my father's behaviour and she did nothing to stop him. This has only put more fuel onto the burning embers of anger and emotion that have been smouldering all of these years.

I have now started to have counselling by a woman who is a survivor herself. It has taken me two years to find the help that I needed. I am sure that if advertising could be made more widespread about organisations, then more woman like myself would try to survive and let others know they are not alone. I am sure that this would give them the courage and determination they need to survive.

I'M BETTER NOW

Blood oozes on to my clothes
And drips to the floor
What shall I do now?
I'll sit and wait,
Wait for what?
You're not going to die!
When I start cutting
I often think I want to be dead,
When I've made a mess
I just want to sit and cry.
I cry because I'm scared
Of what others will think,
Just sew me up
And let me go
I'm O.K. now.
Please don't make me face
All those I've let down.
I want to move on
Until the next time,
I don't want friends
They only get hurt.

This poem was written by Jane in 1983, four years before her death from a drugs overdose.

ANON

I am 16 years old and have been cutting myself for 9 years now. It all began when I was 7. I started to cut myself with knives, then one day, in the same year, I purposely cut my hand with a knife and ended up having stitches in Accident and Emergency. I went out of my way to lie to everyone on how I had done it because I was scared of what everyone would say and because of the reaction I would have got off my 'parents'. So, I said that I had cut my hand on a stone, but I know the nurse saw right through me. Since then I've cut myself on a regular basis.

Things got worse when I was 12, I then started on my wrists for a better response. I would cut myself and then bandage my arms because I felt guilty and ashamed. On my 13th birthday I deliberately got myself run over, but as usual it was an 'accident'. I got to the stage where I was cutting myself almost every day.

At the beginning of this year, I started overdosing on Paracetomol, but without telling anyone: that was when social workers got involved again in January, though my doctor and school convinced them everything was O.K. and I had cut myself on brambles - not that they believed me. In May I got two new social workers whom I hated. I ran away from home and in July I tried to hang myself. A friend found me and encouraged me to see my doctor. Social services didn't get involved because I told them I had a neck scarf on too tight. My doctor referred me for treatment but I wouldn't go and he has now told me that because my suicide attempt was half hearted, he is going to speak to my social worker.

All this began because my Mother was always very violent towards me and so were a lot of her boyfriends. Then when I was 12 and until I was 14, a man used me sexually. I think the thing that really affected me was my relationship with my Mother. I still live with my Mother and even though she has not been violent towards me since the beginning of the year, I still hate her and I don't trust her. If I had not cut myself, I don't think I would be alive now, or at least not relatively sane.

The only useful help was talking to my doctor. Even though I can see his point of view, I feel he has betrayed my trust. Social services have been the least useful; they just think I'm disturbed and I am 'uncooperative' as I find it all a game. Funny game! I am frightened of what is going to happen next but it does not really bother me if I'm alive or dead.

ABUSE

There appeared before me
A strange, dark shadow.
It oozed nightmare,
Spitting out venom in its mutterings and groanings,
Irradiating the air with a poisonous aura.
It was a thing of pure wretchedness,
Of inherent, undiluted evil.
It sought to share its inner turmoil.
Its finger - like extremities reached out.
It almost seemed to hesitate,
But then it gathered new momentum.
At its touch, beautiful creatures fell, dead,
Or lay, when it had gone, writhing in internal pain.
It saw, or seemed to, and faltered again.
Then it began once more to reach out
And touch and maim.
How could it?
How could something be so pitiless, so cruel?

And then it turned to me.
I became hypnotised by its icy gaze
And I felt empty, as if I had lost a part of me.
It seemed suddenly familiar to me,
But I couldn't think where I'd ....

It was coming towards me,
Advancing with gritted teeth
And malice in its gait.
I screamed in terror
And I raised the mallet high.
The creature drew nearer.

It was repulsive; it made my stomach lurch.
It leered and grimaced at me.
For a brief moment I thought it was trying to communicate.
My confusion welled up inside me,
Burning, driving, fuelling my strength.
It was a violence I had never known in myself before.
It frightened me.

And now the desire to destroy it was overwhelming.
The creature clung to my feet.
I struck
And as the mallet fell,
I saw a single tear staining its deformed face
And then I didn't know if I was killing it
From terror, hate, or to put it out of its own misery.
As the weapon hit full force,
The sinews shattered in my own arm.
At once I was whole again,
Alone, exhausted and in pain.
The monster had slithered back to its birth place
And had become, once again,
The dull ache that was my soul.
It huddled in a tight ball in my stomach
And breathed.
It would return.

'Cutting Up'

ALEX BENJAMIN

The first time was when I was twelve. I stole a knife from the kitchen drawer , took it to school with me and at break time I traced tiny bloody marks across my wrist and arm. I then cleaned myself up, took a couple of deep breaths and went to my lesson.

This pattern which was to repeat itself over a number of years. It was my secret, a secret which I found deeply shameful. I remember feeling that I would die of embarrassment if anybody found me out.

My cutting would follow a clear pattern which, over the years, I gradually became to recognise. It would begin with a period of intense anxiety which would escalate over a number of days or weeks. When the anxiety peaked, and I felt I could no longer stand it, I would prepare for the inevitable occasion by locking myself in my room and getting out my secret box. Only then would I allow myself to give in to the desire to slash myself repetitively.

I would try to resist for as long as I could as I knew what would happen if I gave in to the longing. I wanted to hurt myself as I knew that the physical pain would relieve the emotional torment I experienced inside.

By the time I started university, I had a secret store consisting of knives, bandages, plasters and disinfectant which I kept hidden from sight in a special box. I has a number of knives which I would purchase in town when the craving was too much to bear. All I could think about was the need to cut myself. It was like a compulsion. But, in spite of this desperate element, I felt more in control that I ever had before in my life.

To this day, I don't know why I first decided to cut myself. All I know is that it worked.

SECTION SEVEN

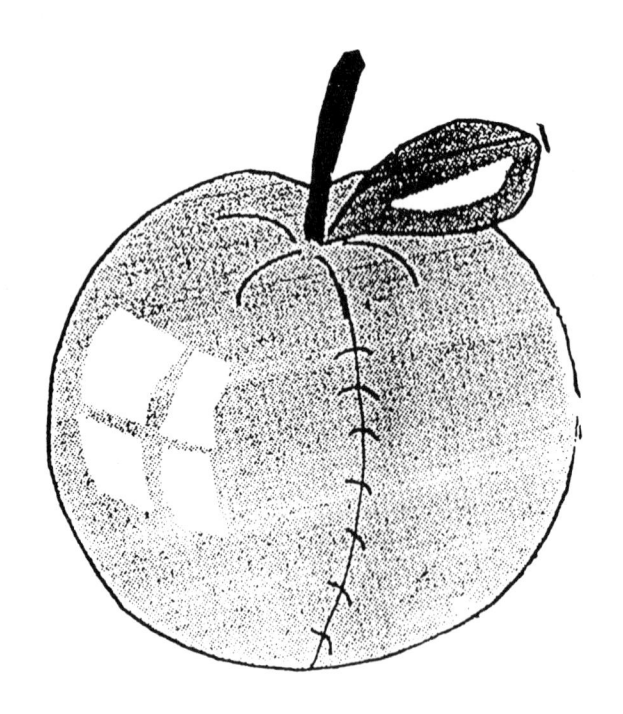

RESEARCH FINDINGS - Preliminary Conclusions and Ideas for Improvement

Preliminary findings from Ashworth Special Hospital

Although research on women who self harm in Ashworth Hospital is preliminary and no firm conclusions have been drawn, interview data conducted by Liebling, Chipchase and Wetton, has so
far identified some of women's stated needs in relation to self harm. Commonly women wished for assistance with expressing feelings and solving problems and wanted a regular listener. A large majority (88 per cent) wanted involvement in planning for their future and 85 per cent wished to have positive goals in their treatment. Women felt a change in environment, i.e. to be in a regional secure unit, or in a more relaxed atmosphere would reduce their need to self harm; although the highest demands were to be at home or live with the family, or to have their own flat.

Liebling and Chipchase (94) say that "the therapeutic needs of women who harm themselves in Ashworth Hospital are currently not being met." They have set up a therapeutic group for women who self harm, which "takes a cognitive-behavioural approach and looks at skills building and mutual support. It also draws on some femininist principles shown to be effective in reducing women's distress." They say how, "the emotional empowerment in women is essential" and go on to talk about the importance of improved education of nursing staff in taking a more positive approach to women who self harm.

A group such as this may be useful in giving women the time and space to voice their feelings and concerns, although it remains to be seen whether any arising suggestions about women's needs will be heard and acted on by hospital authorities. Yet to achieve any real 'emotional empowerment', women will need to have evidence of authorities really acknowledging the difficulties being faced: by bringing abusive staff to justice, and developing a service which is truly sensitive to women's needs. This would ensure that there were enough good, professional staff available for women to talk to, who would support them in becoming involved in their treatment and future plans.

Women's Experience of Services

The Bristol Crisis Service for Women through their research project have surveyed the experiences of 76 women who had come in contact with health and social welfare services in respect of their self injury or related issues. Women were asked to comment on how helpful these services had been. The most commonly mentioned service providers were psychiatrists and psychiatric hospitals, G.P.s, Accident and Emergency departments and counsellors or therapists ('counsellors' and 'therapists' came from a variety of disciplines and it was not always possible to identify the profession of someone who had provided counselling, for example some community psychiatric nurses and psychologists are probably represented in the figures and comments given for counsellor/therapists). Some women had also seen social workers or clinical psychologists. The table below shows numbers of women coming into contact with these services and whether they were generally satisfied, dissatisfied or partially satisfied by the service they had received.

Service Used	No. attended.	Percentage satisfied.	Percentage dissatisfied.	Percentage partially satisfied.
Casualty	16	6	69	25
G.P.	24	37	46	17
Psychiatrist	34	15	82	3
Psych. Hosp. (Inpatient)	23	4	96	0
Psychologist	9	22	78	0
Counsellor/ Therapist	30	63	30	7
Social Worker	10	20	70	10

The Women's Crisis Service go on to state the "high degree of dissatisfaction with many services, with the exception of those who give counselling/psychotherapy." A MIND report on services states that "Enormous sums are being spent on maintaining services that most women do not want. They are being fobbed off with prescriptions for psychotropic drugs... They are subjected to treatments like forced feeding and ECT, which many women find abusive." The report goes on to say that resources should be redirected into the services women want. From my own work and from the research undertaken by the Crisis Service, particular services being called for include: support of a non medical nature such as 24 hr. crisis lines; drop in facilities; crisis houses; free counselling; support/self help groups; and childcare provision. From their survey, The Women's Crisis Service have highlighted other areas of need which women have asked for:

1. Counselling especially for young people on self harm and abuse issues. Again, young people are usually asking for non medical support and help of an 'informed kind' and want more understanding from those who are already acting as carers. A few women have said that life might have been very different if they had been given a counsellor to speak to when they were young. One woman said, "I think every school should have a counsellor to pick up on this sort of thing."

2. More reliable and regular counselling and not to have appointments suddenly cancelled. Women have asked for more counsellors with direct experience, or with some in depth understanding. Some women feel it is necessary to be given a phone contact number if things get too difficult. Also being asked for is 'face to face' counselling at night, or at any 'bad ' time.

3. Support networks and groups where women can share experiences without fear of being judged or punished for their actions. Groups need to be regular and frequent - once or twice a week.

4. Counselling groups on personal losses such as miscarriage, abuse and after sexual attack. The hope is that groups would run a couple of times a week.

5. A sound proof room where women could go to 'scream and cry'. This might be within a drop-in centre or somewhere 'safe' and supportive.

6. Education and training for professional and medical staff on this issue. Women are asking for staff to have listening skills and hope that training would give professionals a better understanding of some of the underlying causes.

7. Women want to be able to speak with medical staff without fear of being judged, condemned or sectioned.

8. The need for someone to act as an advocate/supporter when going into Accident and Emergency department for medical treatment. Also counsellors on staff teams who would be available to speak to.

Women have a huge amount of knowledge as to what they need, yet few crisis facilities and drop-in centres exist to even begin to fulfil those demands. The gap between what there is and what women need can seem dauntingly huge as the lack of resources extends right through to voluntary agencies who provide some free counselling places. These agencies are in short supply and quickly become over subscribed, often able to give little more than short term support. It cannot be argued that good counselling and support services are expensive; they would be much cheaper and more effective in the long term than this continual 'patching up' of women's distress. The question is, can we really afford to go on saying 'this is how it is?' We need to make a shift away from this stuckness to create some changes.

I was a founder member of the Bristol Women's Crisis Service before leaving to set up as a private consultant, although many thought the Crisis Service would never get off the ground - because of what it would cost, and because it was thought that self harm was not a huge issue. Through hard campaigning work and publicity we proved that self harm affected many women and our service was badly needed. In this way we found sponsors who gave us money to get started. After that we managed to fund our first paid worker and now the service has been given money to research the whole area of self harm and discover what is needed. I truly believe that anything is possible if enough people share a similar vision. Now my own personal dream is of a spread of safe houses for women throughout the country where women could choose to take time out from the world when feeling vulnerable. These would include creche facilities where women would be able to leave their children in safe keeping yet be able to see them whenever they wished. I would also like to see more counselling services which specialise in self harm and therapy centres which could offer various counselling and alternative therapies. So often as it is now, services for women are spread over large areas and have little information about each other. If a few of those who worked under the same principles were consolidated under one roof, they would not only be more accessible but their running costs would be reduced.   Also because organisations are having to compete with each other for funding (sometimes without realising it) these problems could be discussed and shared collectively.

But beyond arguing the costs and practicalities, if attitudes towards women's distress moved away from blaming her 'pathology' and focused on what is 'real' for women, then services such as counselling or therapeutic centres would become necessities rather than seem like distant dreams. Not all possible sources of support are expensive to set up and run. For instance, one user led crisis house run through MIND in Wokingham runs on a budget of as little as £4,000 per year. Similarly self help groups can work with very little outlay and running costs. The important point is that we look creatively at what can be done to make changes happen in favour of what women want.

SECTION EIGHT

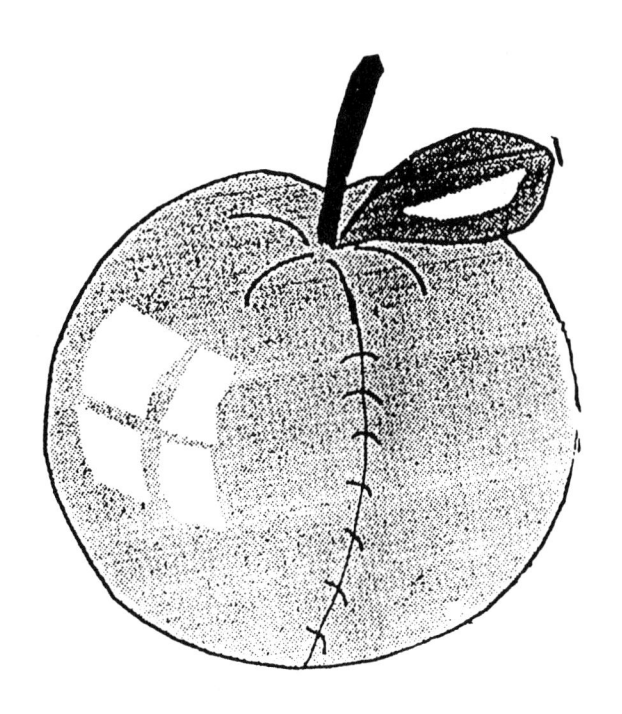

SELF HELP - and what has been useful to women. Rights for women who self-harm

"Having supportive people around who care"

Women have found partners and friends who are accepting especially valuable. Sometimes friends have acted as advocates on women's behalf when going to places such as Accident and Emergency or to see the psychiatrist. Women say it has been helpful to talk beforehand about what needs to be said and what they want from the visit. Afterwards, the 'advocate' can be extremely useful in giving feedback if women are finding it difficult to remember exactly what was said.

"Ending contact with my family"

Sometimes continuing family relationships may further the abusive demands made of women. When working on trying to heal form the past, letting go of abusive ties or creating some physical distance from them may help in releasing old hurts. Similarly, ending hurtful or abusive adult relationships may be part of the process of moving on from continuously finding yourself hurt by someone else - if there is nowhere to go, Women's Aid, single parent projects, support groups or Social Services may be able to help and give support in finding somewhere else.

"Women's groups helped me see my own pain."

"Seeing that other women had been hurt and were expressing their feelings helped me get in touch with my own." "It was good because I felt that at last I fitted in somewhere which was safe."

"Finding other ways to express my anger"

"Hitting pillows in my therapy was too difficult, it didn't seem real. So I joined a self defence class and we hit the hell out of punchbags, which was really good." Several women have become involved in assertiveness training classes, "I learned I had the right to express my feelings and needs." "I found how strong I felt saying NO; I got in touch with my anger and although it was hard at first the instructor was very supportive." Other women have found smashing china useful in expressing their feelings, though I would not personally recommend this exercise as I feel it is easy for women to hurt themselves. Old saucepans are better for throwing onto hard surfaces as they make a noise and can be dented without causing damage. Something else which is useful is rolling up a damp towel and hitting it on a chair or table.

"Drawing or writing on my body instead of cutting"

Using face paints or felt tip pens can be a non damaging way of expressing powerful feelings. Writing words or messages on the parts of your body which you might otherwise injure can put feelings into words. These might then be taken into counselling/therapy or shared with someone supportive if possible. I know of two women who have painted on dolls using bright paint. One woman then tore the doll apart and took the experience along to her therapy. She discovered that she had been trying to destroy her "child-self' was was able to spend time on grieving for this 'lost child' who felt ripped apart.

"Having my own space after sharing a house with friends for a year.

Sometimes the most basic thing that helps is having a place of one's own to live. Homelessness is a growing issue for many women and just having the space to feel 'at home' can alleviate stress from feeling unsafe and insecure. Though some women find that sharing with supportive others helps them feel less isolated. Women's hostels may provide supportive accommodation - though unfortunately there are not enough women only places around.

"Finding people who accept my scars"

"Not feeling that I have to justify my scars to other people but being able to share my self harm with people who I know will not judge me."

"I have shown friends articles about self harm and we have talked about our 'coping mechanisms'
for getting through tough times. I feel better now about wearing short sleeves when I 'm with them and at least I don't have to pretend to be cold in summer!"

"When I found out that other women in my support group self harm it was such a relief not to have to cover up my scars anymore."

"Why should I have to wear long sleeves at work or in public when other people can quite proudly at times show off their sports injuries?"

Louise Pembroke in her book 'Self Harm" has made many suggestions for the 'Rights of self harmers within Accident and Emergency Departments' and has included the right to have scars treated sensitively by medical and emergency staff: "Don't physically humiliate us by leaving us half naked or demanding to see all our scars. Disfigured self harmers require the same sensitivity as patients who are disfigured through surgery or accident." Her excellent book goes on to give useful information about disfigurement.

If there are no support groups locally where these things can be shared, SHOUT Newsletter has news and views from women, so write to them.

"I ask my partner to massage my feet if I'm feeling very ungrounded"

Massage, rather like exercise can help with getting in touch with your physical body. Massage can be soothing but limiting it to "safe" areas like your feet may feel easier than having your body touched. Some women find Shiatsu, where pressure is put on certain energy points in the body, useful in shifting stress; others enjoy aromatherapy oils or try other alternative treatments such as homeopathy.

"Keeping a journal and writing what has happened and how I have felt."

Writing down events, feelings and how these were dealt with can help to build a picture on what triggers the need to self harm. Sometimes women are then able to interrupt the process, for instance by telling a friend they have acted in a hurtful way and saying they feel angry, also by writing down the positive things that have been achieved, no matter how small they may seem. One woman told me that just getting out of bed and making a cup of tea was an achievement for her during a difficult time. After all who is doing the judging on what a successful achievement is? Sometimes just surviving the day should be celebrated as a success!

"Making models out of sculpture, I can put my feelings into the clay"

Any creative physical work can help to alleviate difficult feelings or can be good for grounding when feeling 'spaced out.' I know several women who paint using their hands instead of brushes. A friend of mine pinned a large sheet of paper on the wall and put multi coloured hand prints all over it. But making feelings visible through art work or writing can make them seem more real and women may then want to destroy their work. This is fine, but if possible try first taking the risk of sharing these feelings with someone supportive and then if you wish, 'symbolically' tear them up.

An exercise I have used in groups is to ask women to draw or paint how they see their self harm. Feelings can be given different colours and symbols can be used to represent people or objects which are then shared. This visual exercise can be a good way of identifying otherwise unseen feelings and concerns.

"Not drinking if I feel self harming"

It is important to avoid alcohol or drugs if you are feeling like hurting yourself. Alcohol and drugs can serve to distance women further from their bodies and injuries may be more physically damaging as there is less pain experienced. If substances are used regularly it is worth finding support in dealing with this through organisations such as Alcoholics Anonymous or drugs projects.

"Finding support for my problems with food has helped me think about what I do to my body generally"

Organisations who deal in problems with food such as the Eating Disorders Association can be a useful way of finding support. Health clinics or Wellwoman may be able to give information on what is available locally. There are also some good books available on this issue such as 'Fed up and Hungry", editor Marilyn Lawrence (Women's Press) and "Eating Distress - Perspectives from personal experience, editor Louise Pembroke (Survivors Speak Out).

"Making a list of the things I need to do and then putting off the things that aren't urgent, stops me from feeling overburdened"

Making priorities of any appointments or important needs and concentrating on fulfilling those. Even deciding to do one thing each day can reduce the pressure of overload.

"I am starting to think about my inner judge who demands punishment"

Think about the voice who is telling you to hurt yourself, and see if you can make a connection between that voice and what you heard about yourself as a child. Maybe in some way you heard that you were 'bad' and needed to be punished, and now your 'inner child' expects the same treatment. All children deserve loving attention; they do not deserve to be hurt or neglected. You do not deserve to be punished for what others have done to you.

Learning to cope with panic attacks and flashbacks

"I am learning what can trigger my panic attacks. Being on my own or feeling overwhelmed by feelings because I am in a situation where I feel out of control and powerless or I'm having a flashback. I have to say to myself 'It's O.K., breathe, you are safe. Then I ring a friend and have a list of things which help me feel better, such as a warm bath or reading a book like 'The Courage to Heal'. Even going for a walk or a run if I cannot stay in helps me."

"When I'm in a panic, I can feel so out of control I think I will die. If I can, I try to stay with my feelings because rationally I know they can't kill me, and as my therapist said, I think about my breathing! Sometimes it helps if I ask myself about the things in my life

I do have control of and I write them down to remind me when I'm anxious - things such as, I have control over what I do to my body. And I remind myself that I have choices; I can choose whether to talk to anyone or not today; I can choose to stay indoors today and keep myself safe."

If you have flashbacks, it can be useful to have things around which bring you back to the present day. Some women stick loving poems and posters around the walls, or have notes which give the date and the age they are now. If your mind is racing, try writing down what is happening to you in your journal or notebook. Remember that you are safe now, now one can hurt you, you are in control.

OTHER THINGS THAT MIGHT HELP

Contacting others and networking

Draw up a list of people you feel able to talk to. If you don't know anyone, try contacting SHOUT newsletter who have contacts and a penpal list, or use the resources list in this book.

Caring for injuries

Always use sterile or clean equipment.
Keeping wounds clean reduces the risk of infection.
Never share sharps with anyone else, otherwise you risk serious diseases such as AIDS or hepatitis.

Find a supportive G. P. who will help you care for your injuries. If you can't find one , ask your local Community Health Council for advice on sympathetic G.P.'S.

If wounds do not need medical treatment, to avoid disfiguring scars, use 'steri strips' to close wounds and keep them dry. These can be bought from chemists; some women have even been able to get them on prescription.

Reducing the self injury and limiting long term damage

Try to reduce the amount you self injure on a gradual basis so that the time and amount you hurt yourself becomes less. Each day that self harm has been avoided needs celebrating. But try not to give yourself a hard time if you do resort to harming - it may well have been the only thing you were able to do at that particular time.

Some women have found ways of relieving the need to harm through something physical which gets them in touch with their bodies. A few women have talked about running their hands under cold water and found this also connected them with physical 'matter' which grounded and soothed. Several women have talked about sitting on the floor with their backs pressed against the wall, or even lying on the floor and stamping their feet on the wall. But at times, something which has a larger impact on one's 'self' is used. One woman used ice cubes which she said "shocked me back into my body, which was what I needed at the time"; to gain the same outcome, another used an elastic band around her wrist which she snapped from time to time.

To begin limiting the damage you do to your body, try declaring certain areas 'injury free' and gradually build up from there.

Giving up self harm

Giving up self harm is not easy and you may feel 'pulled' to use this method of coping from time to time. It may be that you need to find other coping strategies that will replace this need, or you may need to work on the underlying issues first. Again, don't give yourself a hard time if you do resort back to harming as this may simply heighten self blame and the need to hurt yourself.

Through their research project, the Bristol Crisis Service for Women have found several women referring to the importance of increased self esteem, having a belief in oneself and assertiveness in helping them leave self harm behind. "It was not always clear what had helped them develop these, but the influence of friends, book groups and courses etc, were amongst those factors mentioned." Also, changes in life circumstances, or "life crises such as major illnesses or the death of someone close had acted as a catalyst for change". The Crisis Service go on to say how some women have found ways of nurturing their bodies; allowing themselves to receive the care and attention they didn't get as children. Relaxation to avoid self injury was mentioned as was massage, walking, having contact with nature, movement and dance. Some women found some form of spirituality helped them overcome harming.

What might help each woman is a matter of individual choice. Several women have told me how self harm eventually became painful and failed to achieve the same outcome it once had. This happened largely after they had acknowledged and were working through some of the underlying issues. Women have said how difficult this time has been, as this tried and 'trusted' coping mechanism no longer works and they are left with their feelings. Having good support is very necessary, as is having enough inner resources to get you through. Regaining feeling is a necessary part of the healing process; powerful feelings are valuable for healing when they are channelled in positive ways.

For me personally I had been terrified of powerful feelings, especially anger for all my life and I went to an anger workshop; rather bravely I feel! Although I thought I would die of fright, I got so angry in that workshop that I screamed out my fury for a whole afternoon. I must say how surprised I was at the end; I was still alive and no one had sectioned me or labelled me as 'crazy'. In fact everyone else was screaming also and the sound was welcomed as a powerful tool in everyone's healing. No matter what our experience in life, we have all been hurt in some way and have the right to express how we feel and be heard.

Go well on your journey.

Be angry - be powerful - be happy - be free!!

Rights and affirmations for women who self harm

1. I have the right to feel safe and to have a secure home life.

2. I have every right to be respected and not be hurt or abused.

3. I do not have to punish myself because other people have hurt me.

4. I have the right to be angry or upset and to have those feelings heard.

5. I do not have to justify my self harm to others.

6. Other people's judgements of my behaviour are based on their own fears and limitations. I am coping the best way I know how.

7. Others do not have to like what I do to myself, nor do they have to be around when I hurt myself. Each of us have our own needs and ways of coping.

8. I have the right to own my body and be in control of happens to it . I also own my feelings and am responsible for how I deal with them.

9. I am not responsible for how other people deal with their feelings.

10. I have the right to express my distress and given the things that have happened in my life, I should be congratulated for having found a way of surviving.

11. I am in charge of my life. I have the right to say what I do and do not want for myself, now and in the future. I also have the right to change my mind.

12. I am the expert in my own life - no one else really know my reality, and what I feel and need for myself.

13. I have the right to want attention and to ask for support from people who could help - although I realise that people cannot always give me the support I need, I do not have to see this as a rejection of me as a person.

14. I have the right to want a lot of support during difficult times. I am not at fault if existing resources do not meet my needs.

15. I have the right to have helpful information made available to me.

RESOURCES THAT MIGHT BE USEFUL IN FINDING SUPPORT

Groups

Although there are very few support groups for self harm, some women have found support from other groups such as those which run for survivors of sexual abuse and women's organisations. Women's centres may run or know of survivor groups and can give valuable information generally. Some may even support the setting up of new groups by acting as a central contact point. Or they might be able to provide room space for meetings. Mental health groups such as MIND already operate some drop in facilities, run user groups, and can give advice on what is available locally in the way of support.

Counselling

Some health clinics and G.P. practices can refer people for counselling and some have a counsellor within their practice. G.P.'s may be able to refer women on to counselling groups. It is also worth asking at places such as Wellwoman, voluntary agencies and Citizens Advice Bureaux to see what services are on offer. 'One advantage with voluntary organisations is greater confidentiality; the fact that women have sough help will not be on their medical or employment records' say the Bristol Crisis Service who have recently brought out three very useful booklets on self harm and have listings on how to go about getting help.

RESOURCES

SUPPORT:

Afro-Caribbean Mental Health Association, 35 -37 Electric Ave, London SW9 8JP. Tel:0171 737 3603. Advice and support.

Anorexia and Bulimia Association - Counselling helpline Wednesday evenings and can provide information. Tel. 0181 8853936 Weds 6-9 pm. Contact: Tottenham Women and Health Centre Annex C, Tottenham Town Hall, Tottenham, London N15 4R8.

British Assoc. for Counselling - Information and advice on Counselling and Therapy. Can provide list of local contacts. Send S.A.E.. to 1 Regent Place, Rugby, Warwickshire, CV21 2PJ.
Tel: 01788 578328

Bristol Crisis Service for Women : Telephone helpline for women. Open Fri and Sats 9pm. -12.30am. Tel O117 251119. Also is doing research into women and self harm to increase understanding and look at areas of need. For further information contact: Research Project, The Bristol Crisis Service for Women, PO Box 654, Bristol BS99 1XH.

Childline 0800 1111. 24hr helpline for children and teenagers.

Eating Disorders Association- Support and advice for people with anorexia and bulimia, also their families. Have details of local groups. Helpline: 01603 621414, Mon-Fri 9am-630pm. Sackville Place, 44 Magdalen Street, Norwich NR3 1JU.

NSPCC 0800 800500. Free 24 hr. helpline for abused children, their families and survivors of abuse. Has information on local resources.

"Off Centre" - Free confidential counselling for survivors of sexual abuse and self harm. Male and female 13-25 yrs, living working or studying in Hackney. Survivors group for women is currently running. Contact 0181 985 8566 or 0181 986 4016 Tues 7-9pm.

SAFE   3 Lumley Walk, Amesbury, SP4 7SB. Helpline 01722 410889. Weds - Sun 6-9pm. Support for ritual abuse survivors.

Sheffield Counselling and Therapy Service. Offers face to face counselling for women survivors of sexual abuse. Contact: 44 Daniel Hill, Upperthorpe, Sheffield S63JF. Tel: 0114 2752157.

Samaritans - for local number, dial the operator or look in front section of telephone directory. Survivors of Sexual Abuse - Helpline 0181 890 4732.

Threshold - (Brighton) Initiative for women and mental health. Offers some face to face counselling. Also organises conference on womans mental health, self help groups and produces a newsletter. Contact Threshold, 79 Buckingham Rd, Brighton, East Sussex, BN1 3RT. Tel: 01273 749800

Women Against Rape - King's Cross Women's Centre, 71 Tonbridge St, London WC1H 9DZ. Tel: 0171 837 7509. Counselling, legal advice and support for women who have been raped or assaulted.

Women's Aid Federation, PO Box 391, Bristol BS99 7WS. Tel: 01179 633494. Helpline: 00117 9633542. Advice, help and information for women suffering from domestic violence.

Womens Therapy Centre - (London) Services for survivors of sexual abuse and training for workers Face to face counselling and groups. Contact. Womens Therapy Centre 6-9 Manor Gardens, London. N7 6LA Tel: 0171 281 7879 Mon-Fri, 2-4pm.

SELF HELP AND NEWSLETTERS:

Hidden Scars - A self help group for women who self injure. Contact: Hidden Scars, c/o Greencroft Centre, 42-46 Salt Lane, Salisbury, SP1 1EG.

Nottingham Self harm support network - Trying to support and network women who self harm. Contact Lexi Reed, c/o 109 The Downs Silverdale, Wilford, Nottingham, NG11 7PH.

SHOUT - Womens newsletter on self harm. Issued bimonthly. Organised and produced by women who have experience of self harm, Also has information about support groups - available to subscribers. For further information contact SHOUT, PO Box 654 Bristol BS99 1XH.

Survivors Network (Sussex) - Self help groups and forums for women survivors of sexual abuse. Newsletter for members. Contact P.O. Box 188 Brighton BN1 JW

Survivors Speak Out - A self advocacy organisation for people who have used psychiatric services. Offers contact, information and a quarterly newsletter. Contact: 34 Osnaburgh St, London NW1 3ND Tel: 0171 916 5472

MALE SURVIVORS OF SEXUAL ABUSE - Contacts:

Consent - Services for male survivors of sexual abuse and rape. Contact: 19 Brabner

House, Wellington Row, London E2 7BE. Helpline 0171 613 5486 Tue & Fri 7-11pm Off. 0181 678 0433

Survivors (Wilts) Counselling and info on local support groups for men recovering from sexual abuse. c/o Health Matters 47a Fleet Street, Swindon SN1 1RE (Postal address only). Helpline Wed 7.30-9.30 Tel 01793 480304

TRAINING:

A.S.H.E.S - (Abuse and Self Harm, Experience of Survival) Training on self harm and sexual abuse issues. Training packages offered. Led and facilitated by survivors who have had several years experience of working with professional agencies and voluntary organisations. Contact: 0117 9711844 or 0117 414258.

Bristol Crisis Service for Women - See support.

Survivors Speak Out - Training and skill sharing. Have run training sessions and events for survivor trainers and actively promote the training of professional people by survivors. See Support.

USEFUL CONTACTS:

42nd Street - (Manchester) is undertaking research on suicide and self harm in young people aged between 15 and 25. Contact: Helen, 42nd Street, 4th Floor, Swan Buildings, 20 Swan St, Manchester M4 5JW. Tel: 0161 832 0170

MIND - (National Association for Mental Health), Granta House, 15/19 Broadway, Stratford, London E15 4BQI. Tel: 0181 519 2122. Legal advice Line 2-4.30pm Mon, Wed, Fri. Information line 0181 522 1728.
MINDlink - Information and contact network. Run through Mind, though is part of the broader user movement in putting forward suggestions for MIND policy and campaigns. In contact with user organisations and Statutory bodies. Contact: MINDlink Co-ordinator, address above.

WISH (Women in Special Hospitals and Secure Units) 25, Horsell Road, London N5 1XL. Tel: 0171 - 7006684.

USEFUL READING:

RADICAL FEMINIST THERAPY Bonnie Burstow. Sage, 1992. (Chapter 10 Self mutilation)

SELF HARM - Louise Roxanne Pembroke, Editor. Cost: £6.60, (£4.50 for survivors) price includes postage and packing. Available from Survivors Speak Out, 34 Osnaburgh Street, London NW1 3ND.
Three Booklets on self harm are now available from the Bristol Crisis Service for Women: 1. Understanding Self Injury. 2. Self Help for Self Injury 3. For Friends and Family.

Diane Harrison

BIBLIOGRAPHY

<u>BOOKS</u>

Barry, K, FEMALE SEXUAL SLAVERY. (1979) New York University Press. New York. 23.

Bettleheim, B, SYMBOLIC WOUNDS. (1955) Thames and Hudson. London.

Boneparte, Marie, FEMALE SEXUALITY. (1953) International Universities Press Inc, New York. 62, 76 - 115.

Breggin, Peter, TOXIC PSYCHIATRY. (1993) Harper Collins, London. 290 - 297.

Briere, Hohn, N, CHILD ABUSE TRAUMA. (1992) IVPS (Interpersonal Violence: Practice Series, SAGE Publications, London. 35 - 51.

Brier, J and Conte, J, AMNESIA FOR ABUSE IN ADULTS MOLESTED AS CHILDREN. (1987) Journal of Traumatic Stress. 49.

Brinton Perera, Sulvia, DESCENT TO THE GODDESS (1981) Inner City Books, Toronto, Canada. 54 - 55.

Burstow, Bonnie, RADICAL FEMINIST THERAPY. (1992) Sage, London. Chapter 1: 'Self Mutilation'.

Busfield, J, MANAGING MADNESS. CHANGING IDEAS AND PRACTICE. (1986) Hutchinson, London. 33.

Chesler, Phyllis, WOMEN AND MADNESS. (1972) Allen Lane, New York. 31, 36 - 38, 40 - 55.

Cooper, W. W, ON WOUNDS AND INJURIES OF THE EYE. (1859) John Churchill, London. 47.

Conway, D.J, MAIDEN MOTHER CRONE. (1994) Llewellyn Publications, St Paul, USA. 83 - 90.

Dryden, Windy, INDIVIDUAL THERAPY IN BRITAIN. (1984) Harper and Rowe Ltd., London 26 -27.

Dworkin, A, WOMAN HATING. (1974) Dutton, New York. 74, 24.

Favazza, Armando, R, BODIES UNDER SIEGE. (1987) John Hopkins University Press, Paperback edition 1992, London. 14 -16, 56 - 87, 132, 169, 187, 218-226.

Fossum, M, and Mason, M, FACING SHAME; FAMILIES IN RECOVERY. (1986) 17.

Gage, M. J, WOMEN, CHURCH AND STATE. (1972l Arno Press, New York.

Goffman, Erving, STIGMA. (1968). Penguin Books, London. 30, 123 - 127.

Gray, Miranda, RED MOON. (1994) Element Books Ltd, Shaftesbury, Dorset. 38, 112 - 135.

Hawton K and Catalan J, ATTEMPTED SUICIDE. (1987) Oxford Medical Publications. 20 - 23, 153.

Inglis, Brian, NATURAL MEDICINE. (1979) Wiilliam Collins and Sons Co Ltd., London.

Johnstone, Lucy, USERS AND ABUSERS OF PSYCHIATRY. (1989) Routledge, London. 102 - 126.

Jung, Carl, MAN AND HIS SYMBOLS(1964) Aldus Books, London. 23, 154.

Lowen, Alexander, NARCISSISM - Denial of the true self. (1985). Macmillan Publishing Co, N.Y. N.Y. 13 - 24, 160 - 178.

Middleton-Moz, Jane, 'SHAME AND GUILT - Masters of Disguise.' (1990) Health Communications Inc, Washington USA. 64 - 65.

Miles, R, THE WOMEN'S HISTORY OF THE WORLD. (1989) Paladin, London.

Miller, Dusty, WOMEN WHO HURT THEMSELVES. (1994) Basic Books, New York,, 10022-5299. 42 - 98, 224.

Millett, Kate, SEXUAL POLITICS. (1993) VIRAGO, LONDON, 178 - 205.

Nelson, Annabelle, THE LIVING WHEEL (1993) Samuel Weisler Inc, York Beach, ME 03910. 9, 22 - 47, 80 - 81.

Noble, V, UNCOILING THE SNAKE; ANCIENT PATTERNS IN CONTEMPORARY WOMEN'S LIVES. (1993) Harper Collins, N.Y. p. 69.

Orbach, S, HUNGER STRIKE. (1986) Fontana, London. 32, 86.

Sayers, Janet SEXUAL CONTRADICTIONS. (1987) Virago Press Ltd, London. 15 - 40.

Schaef, A.M., WHEN SOCIETY BECOMES AN ADDICT. (1992) Thorsons, London. p. 13.

Showalter, E, THE FEMALE MALADY. (1987) Virago, London. p. 11.

Shuttle, P and Redgrove, P, THE WISE WOUND. (1994) Harper-Collins, London. 56, d83 - 86d, 132 - 144, 174 - 249.

Somerset, I.J., SELF INFLICTED CONJUNCTIVITIS. (1945) British Journal of Opthalmology 29: 186 - 204.

Somerville-Large, L.B.c SELF INFLICTED EYE INJURIES. (1947) Trans Opthalmological Soc, U.K. 67: 185 - 201.

Ussher, Jane, WOMEN'S MADNESS, MISOGYNY OR MENTAL ILLNESS? (1991) Harvester Wheatsheaf, Hertfordshire. 20 - 29, 87, 141, 164, 251.

Walsh, B.W and Rosen, P. M, SELF MUTILATION: THEORY RESEARCH AND TREATMENT. (1988) Guildford Press. 5 - 9.

Welldon, Estella, MOTHER MADONNA WHORE. (1988) THE GUILDFORD PRESS, LONDON.
33-34.

Wolf, Naomi . THE BEAUTY MYTH. (1990) Vintage, London. 56 - 57, 150 - 243.

ARTICLES used

Blake-White, Jill and Kline, Christine M. "Treating the Dissociative Process In Adult Victims of Childhood Incest.' (1985) Taken from: The Journal of Contemporary Social Work, Social Casework: Family Services, America. 390-492.

Blessing, Shana, R. 'Self Inflicted Violence (SIV): Perspectives of Women's Self Injury.' From the Seventh International Conference on Multiple Personality Dissociative States, Nov 10, 1990. Article c/o THE CUTTING EDGE, P.O. Box 20819 Cleveland Ohio 44210.

Bradbury, Eileen, M.D., 'The Psychology of Aesthetic Plastic Surgery'. Aesthetic Plastic Surgery Wed Apr 13 09:25:02 1994 Springer Vertag 848.

Briere, John, 'The Long-Term Clinical Correlates of Childhood Sexual Victimisation.' Article taken from the New York Academy of Sciences, vol.528, Aug 12, 1988. 327 -

334.

Briere, John, 'Post Sexual Abuse Trauma." Journal of Interpersonal Violence, Vol 2, No4, Dec 1987. 367 - 369.

Duggan, C Power, M. MacLeod, A. 'Self Injurious Behaviour in Special Hospital: An Intervention Study using Dialectical Behaviour Therapy, Unpublished Study focusing on Rampton Special Hospital.

Gorman, Janet, "Traumatic Memories.' Article in Open Mind magazine April 1994, no.68.

Kreitman and Dyer James A. T. "Suicide and Parasuicide' (1981) Medical Education International Ltd. Nursing and Depression: Nursing 30, 1313.

Liebling H and Chipchase H, 'A Study on the Problem of Self Harming Behaviour in Women in Ashworth Hospital' (1994) Unpublished research findings. p. 75.

McLoughlin, Yvette, ' The Female Body as a Site of Resistance - In the Case of Self Harm.' Dissertation (1993) 73, 79.

Pembroke, Louise, 'Surviving Psychiatry' Published in Nursing Times magazine, December 4, 1991, vol 87, no 49.

Potier, Moira, 'A. 'Giving Evidence; Women's Lives in Ashworth Maximum Security Psychiatric Hospital.' Taken from Feminism and Psychology, 1993 Sage, London. Vol 3(3): 335- 347.

Wise, Mary Louise, 'Adult self injury as a Survival Response in Victim-Survivors of Childhood Abuse.' Journal of Chemical Dependency and Treatment. 1989. 3, 15, 16 - 17, 185 - 201.

Wylie, Mary, Sykes, 'Trauma and Memory.' Networker, September 1993, 42 - 43.

AUTHOR'S NOTE

I am happy to receive written comments about this book. Please send a S.A.E. to me c/o Good Practices in Mental Health, if you wish for a reply. I am open to invitations to discuss the book or to do further training (see A.S.H.E.S in the resources section). However, I do not have time to enter into correspondence with practitioners on individual cases or on the writing of dissertations.

Notes on the cover picture, by the artist

This photograph was originally taken as part of a series of images called It couldn't happen here. It was a small project I was working on in the summer of 1993 about domestic violence. I am a survivor of domestic violence and it had taken me a few years before I could begin to feel ready to do something photographic relating to the experience.

For a few years it had always been in the back of my mind that I should do something. However, I did not want to go and photograph women in refuges and women with bruises because I felt it would be just another lot of documentary photographs that would bring out the voyeur in everyone. The points about why it was happening would be forgotten in the audience's desire to see what a battered woman looked like. I also did not want to use the phototherapy approach.

Like a lot of good ideas the solution came to me late one evening: that I should use a metaphor for a woman. To me the most blatant one was that of the apple in the Garden of Eden; that apple is a symbol of evil women who tempt men. It is associated with women's society. The apple also appears in Greek mythology in the Judgement of Paris, the mortal son of King Priam of Troy. Paris was the one asked by Zeus to settle a dispute between Hera, Athena and Aphrodite about who of the three was the most beautiful. The prize was a golden apple which Paris awarded to Aphrodite. In effect this was the first beauty contest, and women were being judged purely upon what they looked like.

My apple is not golden. It would not be given to the winner. No one in conventional, patriarchal art history would choose it, and it would be discarded in the same way as women who have been beaten and abused are discarded. A common phrase is 'one bad apple can spoil the whole bunch.' Survivors of domestic violence can be treated this way by society, as if by admitting to their existence society itself will be spoiled.

I was trying to create powerful images that which would evoke a gut reaction in people on first sight. I hoped to communicate with people on the subconscious level, even if they were not aware of the intentions I had while making the images. At the same time I wanted to communicate with people who have had similar experiences: to express feelings which occur but which are not always easy to explain in words. In fact I needed to express feelings that go far beyond words, that work on different levels of communication.

The images were shot in domestic surroundings using windfall apples from the tree in the garden and basic light and materials. I felt that to use a studio and to make clean aestheticised prints would just be propping up what my images are against; the squeaky-clean conformity of patriarchal artistic conventions.

The image itself is one to ponder on. Is this apple quickly sewn up to stop us seeing what is inside? Is it sewn so we cannot see what has happened? Is what is on the inside now the same as before the incision was made or has something unwanted been forced in there? The apple will not be the same again - it is damaged goods - and who will want it in a society which discriminates against things which are different from the norm? Will the scar heal? Will the inside mend? Will the scar fade? Will there be some trace of it inside even if the outside looks fine? Will it be strange fruit for the rest of its life? Will it be ever be accepted or will it be just left on the compost heap of life to rot? By extension, all these questions apply to women's roles in society.

To the window cleaner who came round while I was shooting in the garden and asked: 'What are you up to luv? That's a nice camera, is it your boyfriend's?' Well, now you know.

I survived and others can too.

REGAN NOVEMBER 1994